EXERCISE IDEAS

for Conditioning on the Ball

edited by
Jules Vega

VISUAL HEALTH INFORMATION
Tacoma, WA

Cover design by Roxanne Carrington
Publication design and layout by Bethany Maines
Illustrations from the libraries of VHI

10 9 8 7 6 5 4 3

Printed in the United States of America

Publisher's Cataloging-in-Publication
(Provided by Quality Books, Inc.)

Exercise ideas for conditioning on the ball / edited by Jules Vega.
        p. cm.
        ISBN 1-929343-08-6
        ISBN 978-1-929343-08-9

        1. Exercise. 2. Swiss exercise balls.   I. Vega, Jules.

RA781.E895 2005   613.7'1
                        QBI05-200076

VISUAL HEALTH INFORMATION (VHI)
11003 A St. South
Tacoma, Washington 98444-0646

Book Orders: 1-800-356-0709
All Other Inquiries: 1-253-536-4922

CONTENTS

Introduction 1

Chapter 1: Balance & Stability 1

    Beginning 2

    Intermediate 8

    Advanced 15

Chapter 2: Trunk & Abdominals 19

    Beginning 20

    Intermediate 23

    Advanced 26

Chapter 3: Legs 33

    Beginning 34

    Intermediate 37

    Advanced 41

Chapter 4: Arms 49

    Beginning 50

    Intermediate 56

    Advanced 61

Chapter 5: Chest 63

    Beginning 64

    Intermediate 68

    Advanced 73

Chapter 6: Back 75

Beginning 76

Intermediate 81

Advanced 84

Chapter 7: Shoulders 87

Beginning 88

Intermediate 95

Advanced 99

Chapter 8: Combinations 103

Intermediate / Advanced 104

Introduction

This exercise collection has been chosen to meet the needs of the fitness and medical professional. In total, it is comprised of exercise ideas and options that can be used to train the whole body.

This collection is comprised of exercises from the various "kits" produced by Visual Health Information (Tacoma WA). This compilation is representative of most of the exercises that utilize the ball in training. The purpose of the ideas is to provide the reader with options to the exercises they may be employing now. It is not the intent to represent each and every possible exercise option. It is understood that the professional, not the author, is responsible for ensuring that the client's needs, both fitness and therapeutic, will be met by the careful selection of exercises. This is another resource to add to the professional's foundation of knowledge.

The exercises in this collection advance from a position of greatest stability to one of least. Using just the ball, sometimes in conjunction with commercial gym equipment, professionals can use their creativity to meet the needs of their clients in just about any environment. This will make it fun for both the client and trainer, as it will add new and challenging exercises to reinvigorate any program.

It is necessary to provide the reader with the following disclaimer; anyone who attempts to use the exercises in this book without the appropriate training in fitness or exercise, that includes both the client and trainer, will be placing themselves at risk for injury. Consent from a qualified physician or therapeutic professional should be sought when embarking on a new exercise program. The exercises provided are options, *not prescriptions*, and need to be used with the guidance and education of a qualified fitness and or medical professional.

Chapter 1: Balance & Stability

The ball should be properly fitted to the person exercising. While sitting on the ball, the thighs should be parallel to the floor or the hips should be slightly higher than the knees. Correct posture on the ball should be maintained throughout each individual exercise. That means the spine should be in a neutral position, the head erect and the chest held high. As one progresses through the basic positions on the exercise ball, the exerciser will begin to develop greater neuromuscular awareness. This in turn will lead to better postural awareness and control, which will benefit the exerciser during specific body part exercises. As stated earlier, the exercises are presented in a way that will challenge the exerciser progressively.

> Exercises recommended for beginners — These exercises are geared to building a foundation for future work on the ball. Persons who have little or no experience on the ball would be the ideal candidates for this section. It is important not to skip over these as they will ensure that the exerciser will be able to achieve maximal stability for more challenging exercises.

> Exercises recommended for intermediates — This section builds on the previous section by taking the exerciser into positions that require more focus. Once the trainee has completed this section they should be able to move on to the next phase of exercises.

> Exercises recommended for advanced — This section is for high level trainees and athletes. None of these exercises should be attempted without first having mastered the previous two sections. The exercisers who are able to master this section should immediately see an increase in their ability to control the body in space in various sports activities.

Beginning — 25 exercises

Intermediate — 25 exercises

Advanced — 14 exercises

Neck Rotation: Sitting

Gently turn head from side to side.

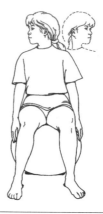

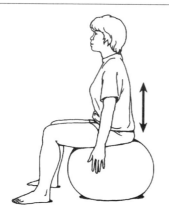

Bouncing: Sitting

Bounce up and down.

Pelvic Tilt: Unweighted

With hands on supports to take weight off spine, gently rotate hips forward and backward.

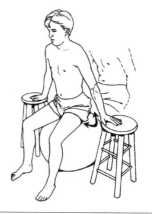

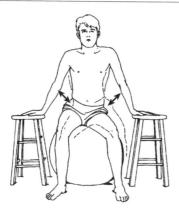

Lateral Pelvic Tilt: Unweighted

With hands on supports to take weight off spine, gently move hips from side to side.

Pelvic Circles: Unweighted

With hands on supports to take weight off spine, gently rotate pelvis clockwise, then counterclockwise.

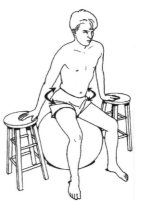

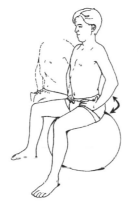

Pelvic Tilt

Gently rotate pelvis forward and backward.

Lateral Pelvic Tilt

Gently move hips from side to side.

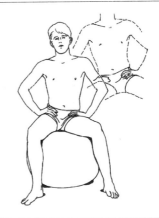

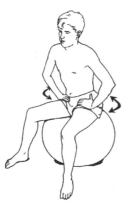

Pelvic Circles

Gently rotate pelvis clockwise, then counterclockwise.

Sitting: Narrow Stance

Sit on ball, feet together, knees at right angles. Maintain neutral spine. Hold.

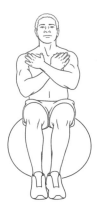

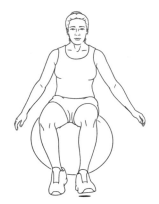

Lateral

Sit on ball, feet together, knees at right angles. Slowly transfer weight to one leg and lift other off the floor. Maintain neutral spine. Hold.

Arm Abduction: Bilateral – Sitting

Raise arms out to side.

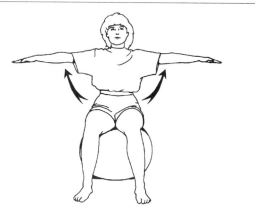

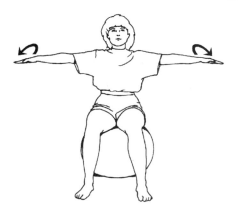

Arm Circles: Bilateral

With arms straight out from sides, make forward circles.

Knee Extension: Sitting

Straighten knee while keeping balance.
Do with or without cuff weights.

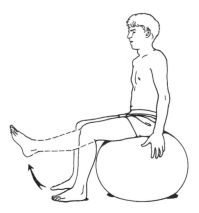

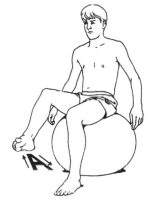

Knee Extension Alphabet Write: Sitting

Straighten knee slightly and trace letters
of alphabet while keeping balance. Do
with or without cuff weights.

Shoulder Flexion: Bilateral – Sitting

Raise arms over head.

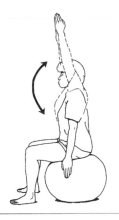

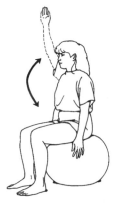

Arm Raise: Alternating – Sitting

Raise one arm above head and
return. Repeat with other arm.

Arm and Leg Raise: Opposite – Sitting

Raise opposite arm and leg and
return. Repeat with other limbs.

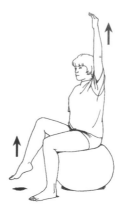

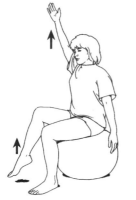

Same-Side Arm and Leg Raise: Sitting

Raise same-side arm and leg and
return. Repeat with other side.

Arm Swing: Sitting

Swing arms forward and backward.

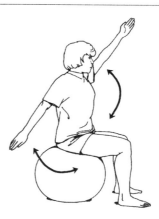

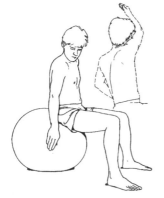

Forward Sitting PNF, Diagonal 1 Flexion / Extension

Sit forward on ball. Raise arm across body and
above head. Follow movement of arm with
head and lean back slightly while reaching.

PNF, Diagonal 2 Flexion / Extension: Forward Sitting

Sit forward on ball. Raise arm from opposite knee across body and reach up. Follow movement of arm with head and lean back slightly while reaching.

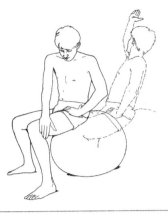

One-Arm Support Opposite-Arm Horizontal Abduction: Kneeling

On all fours over ball, reach up toward ceiling with one arm. Return and repeat with other arm.

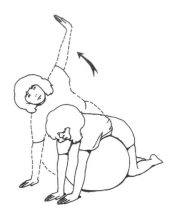

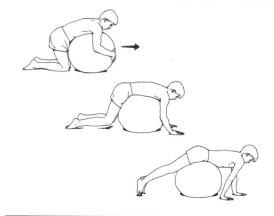

Ball Walk to Toes Touching Floor: Kneeling

Kneeling with stomach on ball, walk forward until toes drag.

Ball Walk to Thighs / Toes: Kneeling

Kneeling with stomach on ball, walk forward until it rests under thighs / toes.

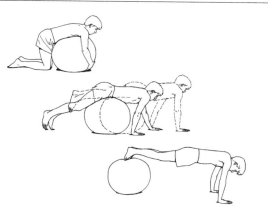

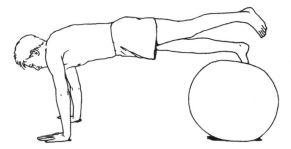

Ball Walk to Toes with Hip Extension: Prone

Walk forward on ball until it rests under toes. Raise one leg from ball. Return. Repeat with other leg.

Ball Walk with Hip Abduction / Adduction: Prone

Walk forward on ball until it rests under thighs. Sweep one leg out to side and return. Repeat with other leg.

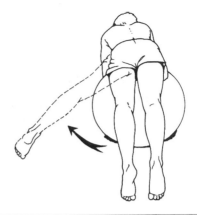

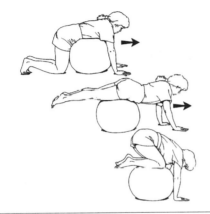

Ball Walk to Double Knee to Chest: Kneeling

Walk forward on ball until it rests under shins. Support weight with hands and roll ball under you by bending knees up to chest.

Ball Walk to "Skier" Position: Prone

With stomach on ball, walk forward until ball rests under shins. Supporting weight on hands, roll ball forward and out to side by pulling with knees.

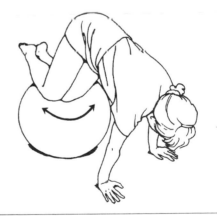

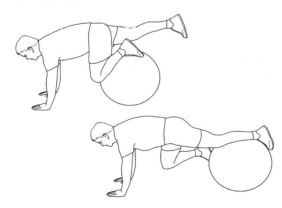

Walkout: with Knee Tuck – Alternating (Gymball)

Roll out to shins. Take one leg off ball. Tuck leg on ball, by bringing heel toward buttock, while straightening other leg. Keeping same leg on ball, alternately tuck / straighten legs.

Side-to-Side Lean: Prone

Lying on stomach over ball, lean
from side to side, catching weight
with same-side hand and foot.

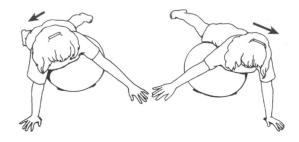

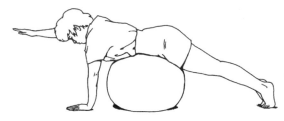

Arm Raise: Alternating – Prone

On hands and toes over ball, raise arm
and return. Repeat with other arm.

Arm Raise: Bilateral – Prone

Balancing with toes, raise both arms.

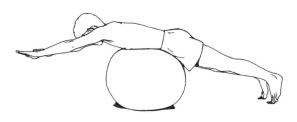

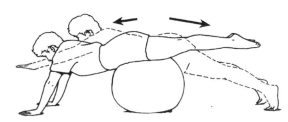

Front-to-Back Rocking: Prone

Lying on stomach over ball, lean forward
and backward, catching body weight
first on hands, then on feet.

Walkout (Gymball)

Walk-roll out to shins, then back.

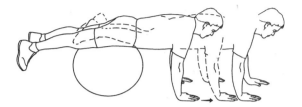

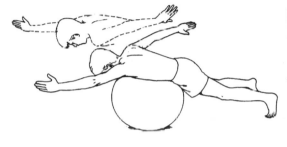

Flexion / Extension: Bilateral Alternating – Prone

Balancing with toes, alternately lift one arm forward and the other backward.

Leg Raise: Alternating – Prone

On hands and toes over ball, raise one leg and return. Do not arch back. Repeat with other leg.

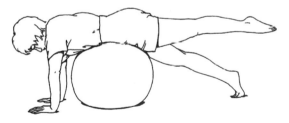

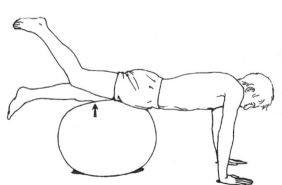

Ball Walk to Thighs with Hip Extension: Prone

Walk forward on ball until it rests under thighs. Raise one thigh from ball. Return. Repeat with other thigh.

Same-Side Arm and Leg Raise: Prone

On hands and toes over ball, raise same-side arm and leg simultaneously. Do not arch back. Repeat with other side.

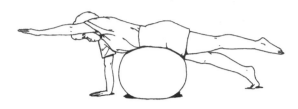

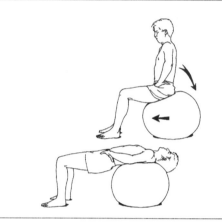

Sitting to Bridging Position

From sitting position, roll forward into bridging position, with ball under shoulders. Do not let hips sag. Return to starting position.

Sitting to Supine Spinal Extension Stretch

From sitting position, roll forward into bridging position with ball under middle of back. Hold.

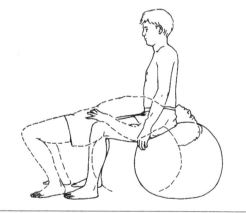

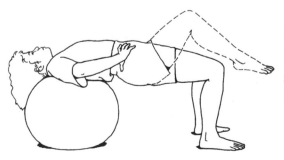

Bridging with Leg Raise

In bridging position with ball under shoulders, raise one bent knee. Maintain balance. Repeat with other leg.

Knee Extension from Bridging

From sitting, walk out to bridge position. Straighten knee while keeping balance.

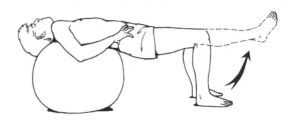

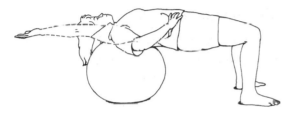

Bridging with Arm Raise

In bridging position with ball under shoulders, raise one arm over head and parallel to floor. Maintain balance. Repeat with other arm.

Bridging with Same-Side Arm and Leg Raise

In bridging position with ball under shoulders, raise same-side arm and leg simultaneously. Do not let hips sag. Maintain balance. Repeat with other limbs.

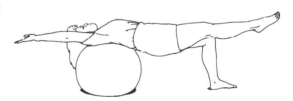

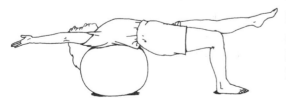

Bridging with Opposite Arm and Leg Raise

In bridging position with ball under shoulders, raise one arm and opposite leg simultaneously. Do not let hips sag. Maintain balance. Repeat with other limbs.

Bridging Leg Sweep Under and Over

With calf and/or heel resting on ball, lift
buttocks off floor. Maintain bridge while
moving other leg over and under leg on ball.

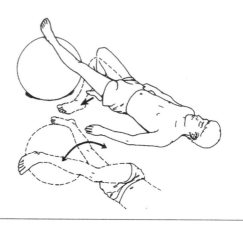

Walkout with Step Over (Gymball/Medicine Ball)

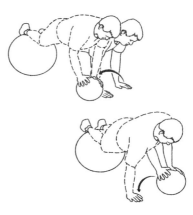

Roll out to shins. Have medicine ball beside hands on floor. Bring one hand then other onto ball. Take one hand then other off ball on other side.

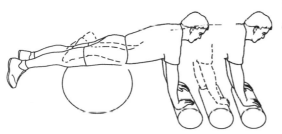

Foam Roller Rollout (Gymball)

On foam roller, walk-roll out to shins then back.

Foam Roller Knee Tuck – Alternating (Gymball)

Hands on foam roller, walk-roll out to shins. Take one leg off ball. Tuck leg on ball toward stomach while straightening other leg. Keeping same leg on ball, alternately tuck / straighten legs.

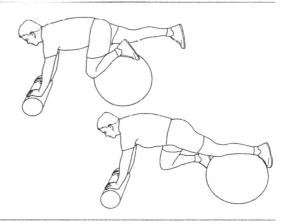

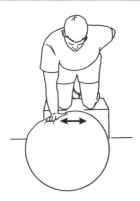

Hand on Ball: Side to Side

Kneel on surface level with top of ball. Place one hand on ball, other hand behind back. Maintain shoulders over ball. Move ball side to side.

Hand on Ball: Front to Back

Kneel on surface level with top of ball. Place one hand on ball, other behind back. Maintain shoulders over ball. Move ball forward to back.

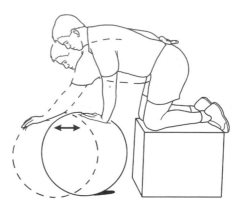

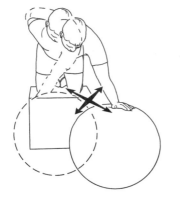

Hand on Ball: Diagonal

Kneel on surface level with top of ball. Place one hand on ball, other behind back. Maintain shoulders over ball. Move ball in diagonal pattern, forward to back, alternating directions.

Hand on Ball: Circle – Clockwise / Counterclockwise

Kneel on surface level with top of ball. Place one hand on ball, other behind back. Maintain shoulders over ball. Move ball in circles clockwise or counterclockwise.

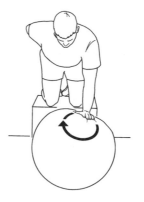

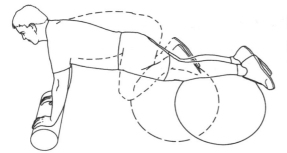

Foam Roller Knee Tuck (Gymball)

Hands on foam roller, walk-roll out to shins. Tuck knees toward stomach, then straighten.

Walkout with Travel (Gymball)

Walk-roll out to shins. Walk hands in semicircle, one direction then the other.

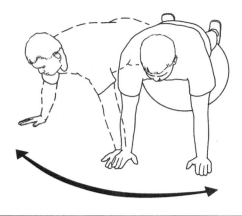

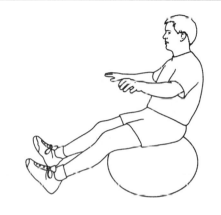

Sit / Balance (Gymball)

Sit and balance on ball. Hold.

"Superman": Prone (Gymball)

Lift both arms and legs off ground while maintaining balance.

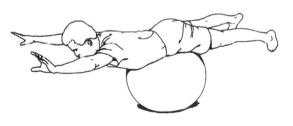

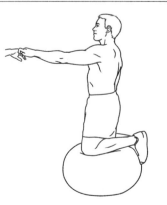

Kneeling: Assisted (Gymball)

Kneeling on ball, maintain neutral spine. Use assistance until secure.

Kneeling (Gymball)

Kneel on ball. Keep trunk upright.

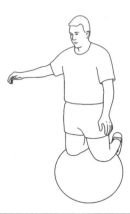

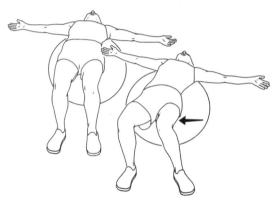

Ball Roll: Supine

Bridge trunk with head, neck, and shoulders supported. Keeping arms extended and parallel with shoulders, roll to one side and hold. Repeat to other side.

Chapter 2: Trunk & Abdominals

This section is designed to target muscles of the back and abdomen. All three sections will help the trainees begin to tone and strengthen the core muscles, which will help them look and feel better. This emphasis on core muscles is one advantage of training on the ball as compared to simply using a bench.

Exercises recommended for beginners — This section will help the exerciser begin to become aware of the abdominal and low back muscles. These exercises should be done in a slow and controlled manner to allow the trainee to feel the contractions of the muscles.

Exercises recommended for intermediates — These exercises should be attempted once the exerciser has become proficient at executing the proper muscular contraction of the targeted muscle groups. The trainee should begin to experience visible muscular and postural changes at this point.

Exercises recommended for advanced — These exercises are very challenging and should only be attempted after mastery of the first two sections has been accomplished. The exercise ball is superior to most other forms of apparatus in that while performing high level movements the exerciser, not the equipment, controls all facets of motion.

Beginning — 12 exercises

Intermediate — 12 exercises

Advanced — 27 exercises

Neck Extension: Kneeling

Extend head up from ball.

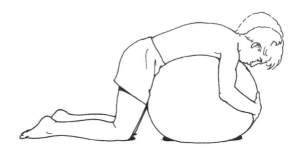

Back Extension: Kneeling

With hands on back of head, extend upper back from ball.

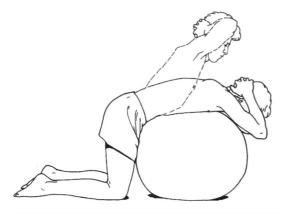

Forward / Backward Roll: Kneeling

Roll ball forward and hold. Return to starting position.

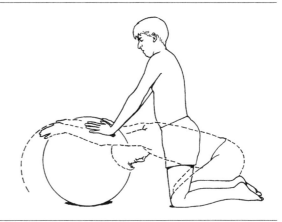

Scapular Retraction: Kneeling

Bend arms and lift, pulling shoulder blades together.

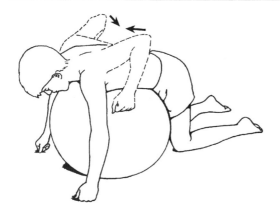

Side-to-Side Stretch: Kneeling

From kneeling, stretch to one side. Hold and repeat to other side.

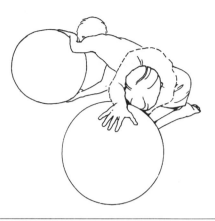

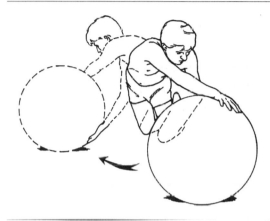

Side-to-Side Roll: Kneeling

Roll ball from side to side, stretching shoulders. Allow arms to bend. Hold on each side.

Horizontal Abduction / Adduction: Kneeling

Keeping arms extended, roll ball from side to side, stretching shoulders. Hold on each side.

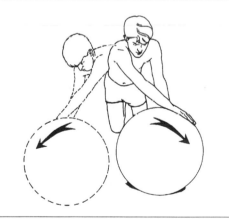

Arm Reach: Forehead-Rest – Kneeling

Reach one arm forward while resting forehead on ball. Return and repeat with other arm.

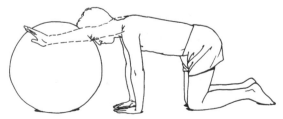

Arm Abduction: Forehead-Rest Unilateral – Kneeling

Reach one arm out to side while resting forehead on ball. Repeat with other arm.

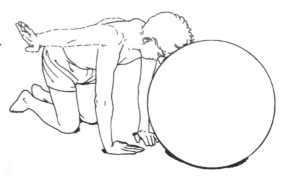

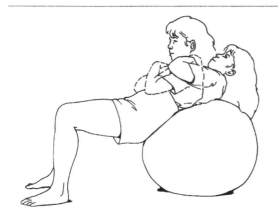

Half Sit-Up: Sitting

From incline sitting position, perform curl-up.

Hip Rotation: Supine

Lying flat on back, rotate legs from side to side.

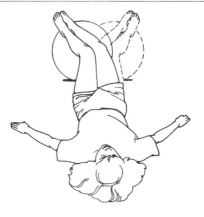

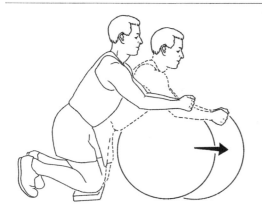

Ball Roll: Basic

With forearms on ball and back straight, begin to roll forward, progressively tensing abdominals. Breathing out, roll back to start position.

Caution: Do not hyperextend low back.

One-Arm Raise with Spinal Rotation: Kneeling

From kneeling, raise one arm while rotating trunk into position shown. Hold, then repeat with other arm.

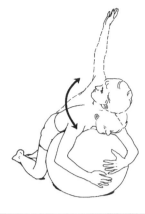

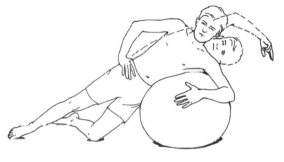

Arm Over Head Stretch: Side-Lying

Reach above head until a stretch is felt. Hold. Exhale as you reach.

Back Extension: Prone

With hands on back of head, lift upper back from ball.

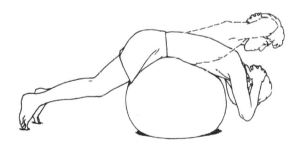

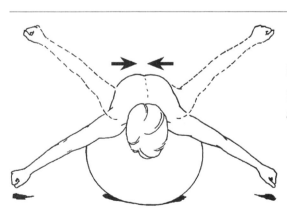

Butterflies: Kneeling

Kneeling on floor with stomach over ball, extend arms and lift to pull shoulder blades together.

Arm Abduction: Forehead-Rest Bilateral – Kneeling

Raise both arms out to side while resting forehead on ball.

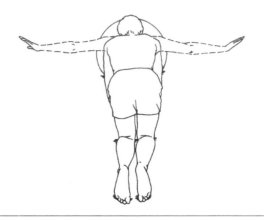

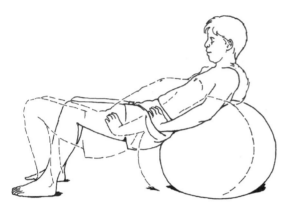

Upper Thoracic Stretch: Sitting

From sitting, slide down ball until shoulder blades come in contact with ball, stretching upper back. Hold.

Middle Thoracic Stretch: Sitting

From sitting, slide down ball until neck comes in contact with ball, stretching middle back. Hold.

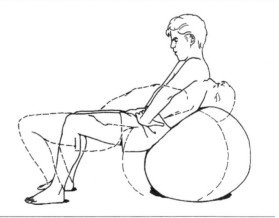

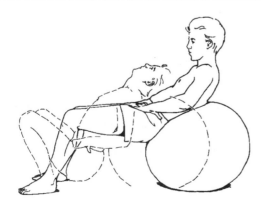

Lower Thoracic Stretch: Sitting

From sitting, slide down ball until buttocks nearly contact floor, stretching lower back. Hold.

Kneeling to Prone Extension Stretch

From kneeling, support body on arms and stretch into dotted position. Hold.

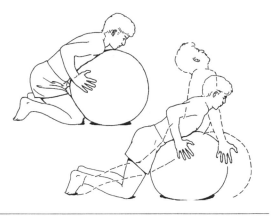

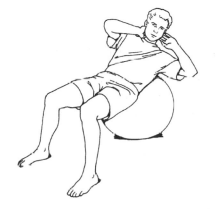

Diagonal Curl-Up: Supine

From reclined position, perform diagonal curl-up, bringing one elbow toward opposite knee. Repeat with other elbow.

Sit-Up: Full – Sitting

From reclined position, perform a sit-up. End with body perpendicular to straightened legs.

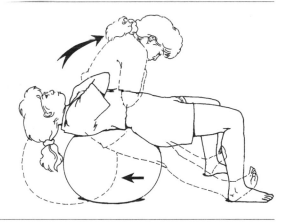

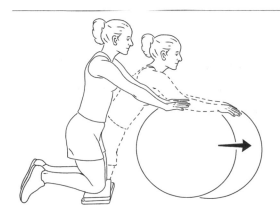

Ball Roll: Intermediate

With hands on ball and back straight, begin to roll forward, progressively tensing abdominals. Breathing out, roll back to start position.

Caution: Do not hyperextend low back.

Ball Walk to "Skier" Position: Prone

With stomach on ball, walk forward until ball rests under shins. Supporting weight on hands, roll ball forward and out to side by pulling with knees.

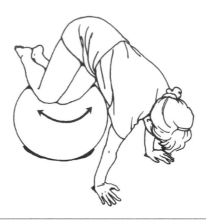

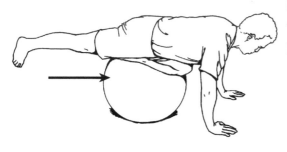

Ball Walk to Single Knee to Chest: Prone

Walk forward on ball until it rests under shins. Move one leg off ball, and pull "ball leg" to chest

Ball Walk to Double Knee to Chest: Kneeling

Walk forward on ball until it rests under shins. Support weight with hands and roll ball under you by bending knees up to chest.

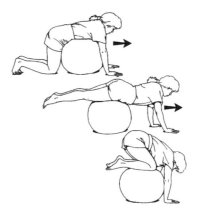

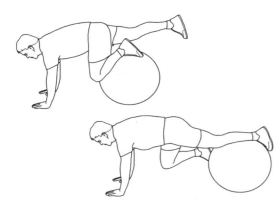

Walkout: with Knee Tuck – Alternating (Gymball)

Roll out to shins. Take one leg off ball. Tuck leg on ball, by bringing heel toward buttock, while straightening other leg. Keeping same leg on ball, alternately tuck / straighten legs.

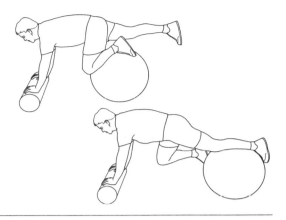

Walkout / Foam Roller Knee Tuck – Alternating (Gymball)

Hands on foam roller, walk-roll out to shins. Take one leg off ball. Tuck leg on ball toward stomach while straightening other leg. Keeping same leg on ball, alternately tuck / straighten legs.

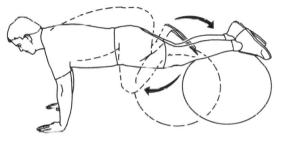

Walkout: with Knee Tuck (Gymball)

Walk-roll out to shins. Tuck knees by bringing heels toward buttocks.

Walkout / Foam Roller Knee Tuck (Gymball)

Hands on foam roller, walk-roll out to shins. Tuck knees toward stomach, then straighten.

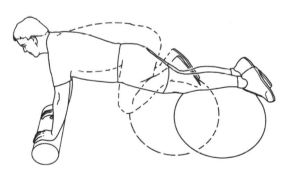

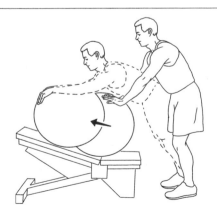

Ball Roll: Incline

With palms on ball, back straight, begin to roll forward, progressively tensing abdominals. Breathing out, roll back to start position.

Caution: Do not hyperextend the low back.

Ball Roll: Advanced

With hands on ball, back straight, knees off the floor, begin to roll forward, progressively tensing abdominals. Breathing out, roll back to start position.

Caution: Do not hyperextend the low back.

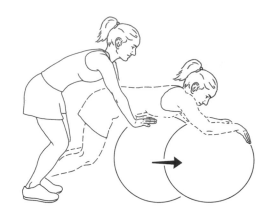

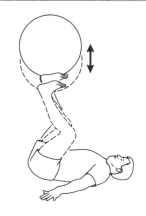

Raise / Lower – Balance (Gymball)

Lie on back with ball on bare feet. Slowly raise and lower ball.

V Sit-Up (Gymball)

Lie on back, legs over ball, hands on floor beyond head. Squeeze ball between calves and thighs. Raise ball and hands to meet in the middle.

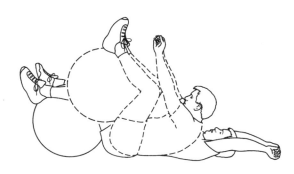

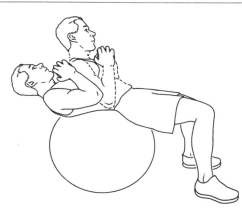

Crunch (Dumbbell)

Hold dumbbell on upper chest, low back supported. Tighten abdominals by bringing ribs toward pelvis until shoulders clear ball.

Crunch: Alternating (Dumbbell)

Hold dumbbell on upper chest, low back supported. Tighten abdominals by bringing right ribs toward left pelvis. Repeat to other side.

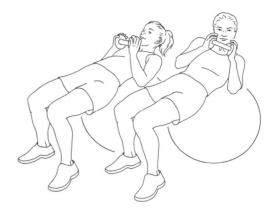

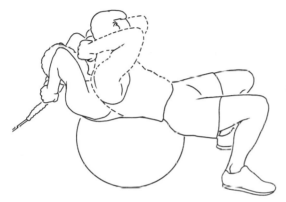

Crunch (Cable)

Grasp rope handle, low back supported. Tighten abdominals by bringing ribs toward pelvis until shoulders clear ball.

Crunch: Alternating (Cable)

Grasp rope handle, low back supported. Tighten abdominals by bringing left ribs toward right pelvis until shoulder clears ball. Repeat to other side.

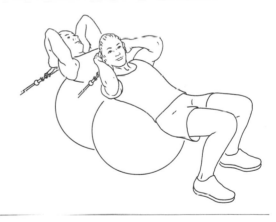

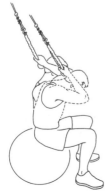

Crunch: Sitting (Cable)

Grasp rope handle over head. Tighten abdominals by bringing elbows toward knees. Only spine moves.

Crunch: Sitting – Alternating (Cable)

Grasp a rope handle over head. Tighten abdominals by bringing left elbow toward right knee. Repeat to other side. Only spine moves.

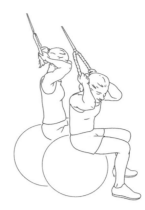

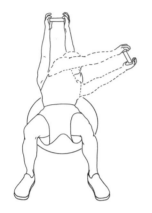

Twist: Supine (Dumbbell)

Bridge trunk, head, neck, and shoulders supported, arms extended overhead holding dumbbell. Rotate trunk to the right, keeping arms extended. Repeat to other side.

Crunch: Reverse

Grasp a stable bar, legs bent, hips at 90°. Keeping abdominals tensed, extend hips then reverse direction.

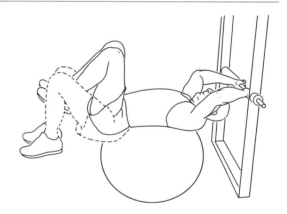

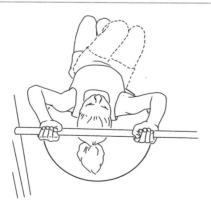

Crunch: Reverse – Alternating

Grasp a stable bar, legs bent, hips at 90°. Keeping abdominals tensed, extend hips then reverse direction by bringing knees toward right shoulder. Repeat to other side.

Straight Leg Raise

Grasp stable bar. Keeping abdominals tensed, extend hips then reverse direction.

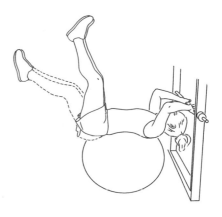

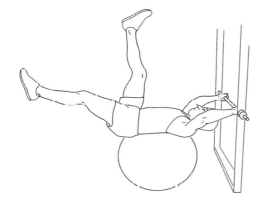

Straight Leg Raise: Alternating

Grasp stable bar. Keeping abdominals tensed, extend one hip then reverse direction. Repeat with other leg.

Wood Chop: Sitting (Cable)

Grasp cable and rotate trunk by bringing hands toward opposite hip. Keep pelvis stable. Repeat to other side.

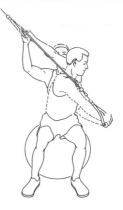

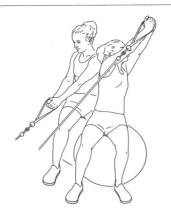

Wood Chop: Reverse – Sitting (Cable)

Grasp cable and rotate trunk by bringing hands above opposite shoulder. Keep pelvis stable. Repeat to other side.

Wood Chop: Reverse – Sitting (Dumbbell)

Grasp dumbbell and rotate trunk by bringing hands above opposite shoulder. Keep pelvis stable. Repeat to other side.

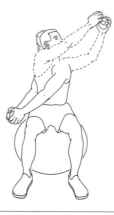

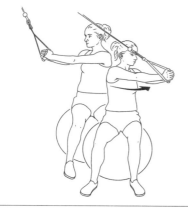

Trunk Rotation: Sitting (Cable)

Grasp cable with arms horizontal. Rotate trunk by bringing arms across body. Keep pelvis stable. Repeat to other side.

Trunk Rotation: Sitting (Dumbbell)

Grasp dumbbell with arms horizontal. Rotate trunk by bringing arms across body. Keep pelvis stable. Repeat to other side.

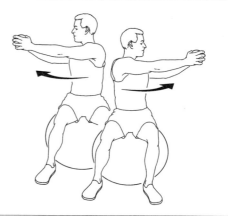

Chapter 3: Legs

This section is designed to work the legs in positions that conventional exercise methods usually do not. A benefit to exercising the legs using the exercise ball is strength gains are realized throughout all the musculature of the lower extremity and not just specific muscle groups. Building stronger legs while using the exercise ball will help to create better symmetry throughout the entire body.

Exercises recommended for beginners — This section is excellent for people who have weak legs and/or orthopedic considerations. Proper care should be taken to ensure that speed of movement and active range of motion are carefully controlled.

Exercises recommended for intermediates — Once the exerciser has become comfortable with the previous section these exercises will challenge more specific muscle groups such as the hamstrings and quadriceps. If using resistance with this section, care should be taken to progress slowly

Exercises recommended for advanced — These exercises are designed to move the athlete through positions that they might encounter in sport or play. At this point the exerciser should have developed the necessary balance and stability to perform these movements safely.

Beginning — 12 exercises

Intermediate — 15 exercises

Advanced — 26 exercises

Bridging with Calves on Ball

Lying on back with calves resting on ball, raise buttocks from floor.

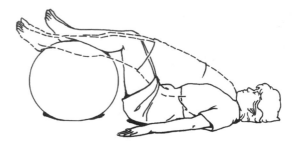

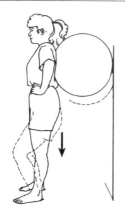

Shallow Squat with Back Against Ball

Perform a partial squat.

Shin Raise with Back Against Ball

Rise up on heels and return.

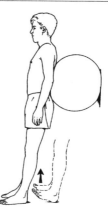

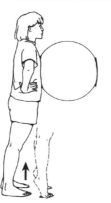

Calf Raise with Stomach Against Ball: Standing

Rise up on toes and return.

Hip Extension Bridging with Calves on Ball

With calves resting on ball, lift hips off floor and return. Keep knees straight.

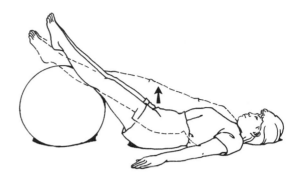

Isometric Adduction: Side-Lying

Squeeze ball between legs.

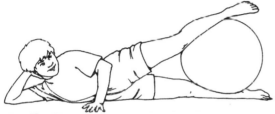

Isometric Adduction: Supine

Lying flat on back, squeeze ball between knees.

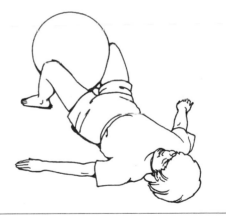

Isometric Abduction: Supine

With ball against wall, press outside of knee into ball.

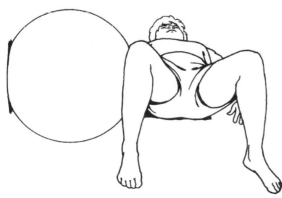

Leg Curl with Hips Flat

With hips and knees bent at 90°
and heels resting on ball, bend knees
so that ball rolls toward you.

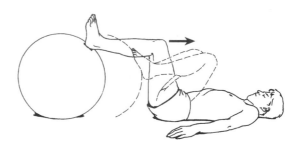

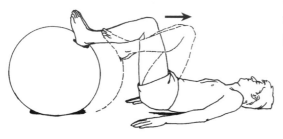

Leg Curl from 2" Bridge

With heels resting on ball and hips lifted 2" from
floor, roll ball toward you by bending knees.

Knee Extension: Sitting

Straighten knee while keeping balance.
Do with or without cuff weights.

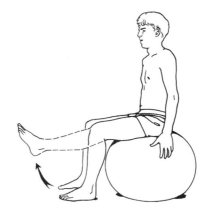

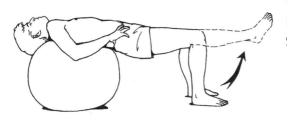

Knee Extension from Bridging

From sitting, walk out to bridge position.
Straighten knee while keeping balance.

Medium Squat

Perform a medium squat as shown.

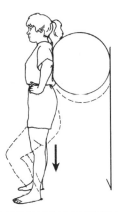

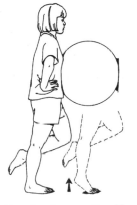

Calf Raise with Stomach Against Ball: Single-Leg

Standing on one leg, rise up on toes and return. Repeat with other leg.

Shin Raise with Back Against Ball: Single-Leg

Standing on one leg, rise up on heel and return. Repeat with other leg.

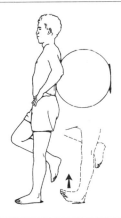

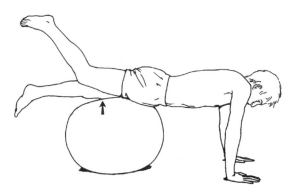

Ball Walk to Thighs with Hip Extension: Prone

Walk forward on ball until it rests under thighs. Raise one thigh from ball. Return. Repeat with other thigh.

Alternating Leg Raise: Prone

On hands and toes over ball, raise one leg and return. Do not arch back. Repeat with other leg.

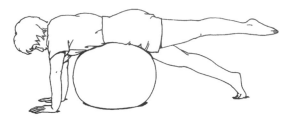

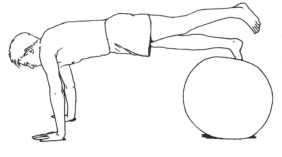

Ball Walk to Toes with Hip Extension: Prone

Walk forward on ball until it rests under toes. Raise one leg from ball. Return. Repeat with other leg.

Ball Walk with Hip Abduction / Adduction: Prone

Walk forward on ball until it rests under thighs. Sweep one leg out to side and return. Repeat with other leg.

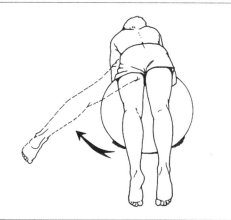

Bridging with Leg Raise

In bridging position with ball under shoulders, raise one bent knee. Maintain balance. Repeat with other leg.

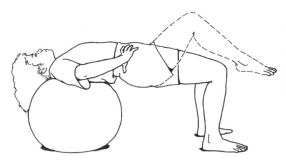

Hip Extension Bridging with Heels on Ball

With heels resting on ball, lift hips off floor and return. Keep knees straight.

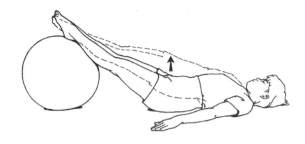

Hip Extension Bridging with Heels on Ball: Slow March

With heels resting on ball and hips off floor, slowly raise one leg 4-6" from ball. Repeat with other leg and perform in a rhythmic fashion. Keep knees straight.

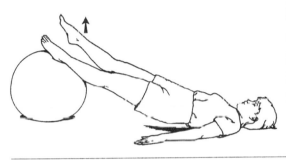

Bridging with Calf on Ball: Single-Leg

With calves on ball and hips off floor, raise one leg from ball and hold. Return to starting position and repeat with other leg.

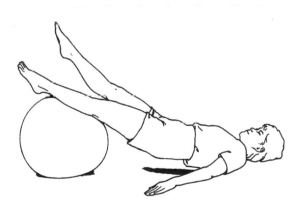

Bridging with Heel on Ball: Single-Leg

With heels resting on ball and hips off floor, raise one leg from ball and hold. Return to starting position and repeat with other leg.

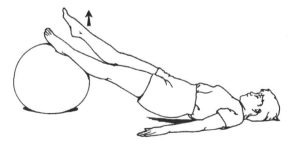

Leg Curl from 4-6" Bridge

With heels resting on ball and hips lifted
4-6" from floor, roll ball toward you
by bending knees. Return to start.

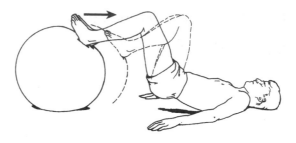

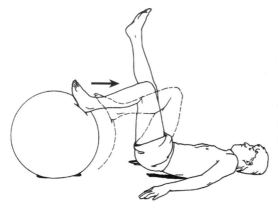

Leg Curl from 4-6" Bridge: Single

With heels resting on ball and hips lifted
4-6" from floor, raise one leg off ball and
roll ball toward you by bending other
knee. Return. Repeat with other leg.

Leg Curl Ball Roll
with Opposite-Knee Extension: Single

Straighten one leg and roll ball toward then away
from you with other leg. Repeat with other leg.

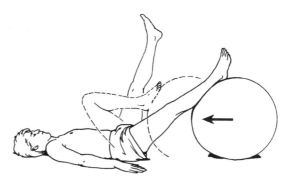

Parallel Squat with Back Against Ball

Perform a deep squat as shown.

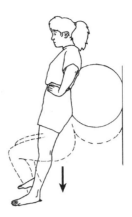

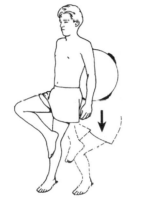

One-Leg Squat with Back Against Ball

Standing on one leg, perform a squat as shown.

Squat: Supported (Dumbbell)

Back straight, bend knees, but do not allow them past toes.

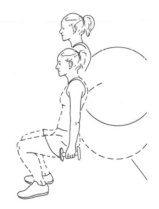

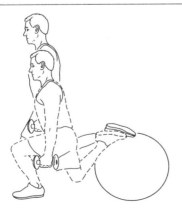

Squat-Split: Foot on Ball

Back straight. Do not allow knees past toes. Repeat with other leg on ball.

Squat-Split: Supported (Dumbbell)

Back straight, bend at knee; do not allow knees past toes. Repeat with other leg forward.

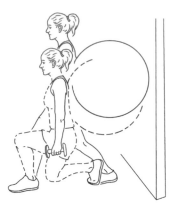

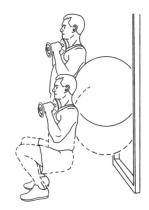

Squat: Supported – Front (Dumbbell)

Back straight, dumbbells at shoulders. Bend at hips; do not allow knees past toes.

Squat: Supported – Lateral (Dumbbell)

Back straight, lean into ball. Bend at knee; do not allow knees past toes. Repeat on same side, legs switched. Repeat sequence on other side.

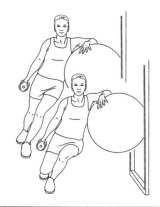

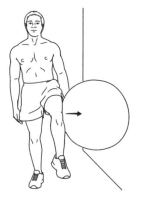

Hip Abduction: Single-Leg Standing

Stand with ball between wall and flexed knee and hip. Press side of knee into ball. Hold.

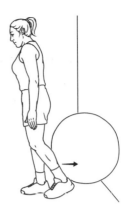

Hip Extension: Single, Standing

Stand with ball between calf of one leg and wall. Squeeze back of leg against ball. Hold.

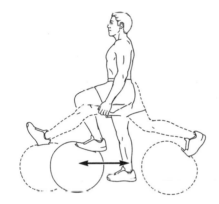

Anterior / Posterior Roll: Single

Standing in neutral posture with one foot on ball, roll ball forward and backward.

Circle Roll: Single

Standing in neutral posture with one foot on ball, roll ball in circles. Repeat with other leg.

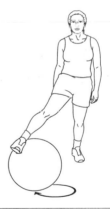

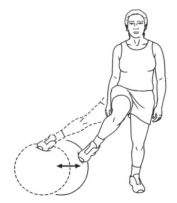

Lateral Roll: Single

Standing in neutral posture with one foot on ball, roll ball out to side, then return.

Calf Raise: Supported (Dumbbell)

Lean on ball and rise up onto toes.

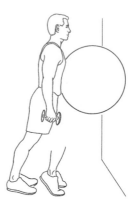

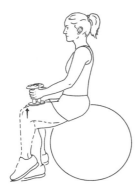

Calf Raise: Sitting (Dumbbell)

Rest dumbbells on thighs and rise up on toes.

Press Leg (Dumbbell)

Hold dumbbells at chest and keep head and neck supported while extending hips and knees.

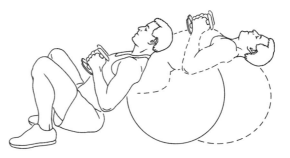

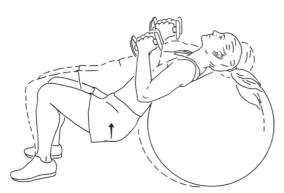

Bridge: Supine (Dumbbell)

Hold dumbbells at chest and keep head and neck supported. Extend hips.

Press Leg: Single (Dumbbell)

Hold dumbbells at chest and keep head and neck supported while lifting one leg and hip. Repeat with other leg.

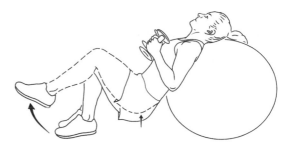

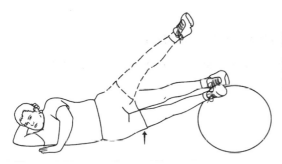

Hip Lift / Leg Lift – Side-Lying (Gymball)

Lie on side with feet together on ball. Support head with hand. Lift hips then lift top leg.

Hip Lift – Side-Lying (Gymball)

Lie on side with feet together on ball. Support head with hand. Lift hips in line with knees.

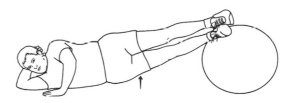

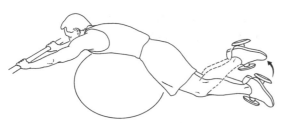

Hamstring Curl: Prone (Dumbbell)

Hold dumbbell between feet and flex knee. Use partner or support if needed.

Hip Extension: Prone (Dumbbell)

Holding support, dumbbell between feet, straighten and lift legs.

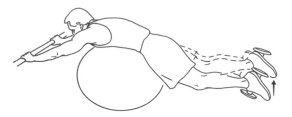

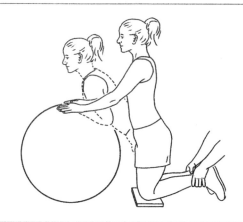

Hamstring Curl: Kneeling

With feet anchored allow body to descend. Tense hamstrings bringing body back to start.

Hip Abduction: Sitting (Cable)

Back straight, knee straight, pull cable out to side.

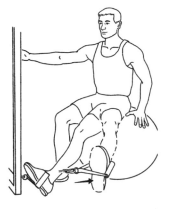

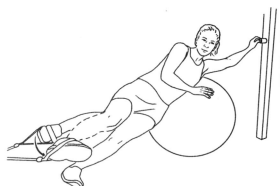

Knee Extension: Single – Side-Lying (Cable)

Extend knee, keeping thigh stable. Repeat with other leg.

Hip Flexion: Knee-Bent, Single – Side-Lying (Cable)

Flex hip, knee bent at 90°. Keep torso stable. Repeat with other leg.

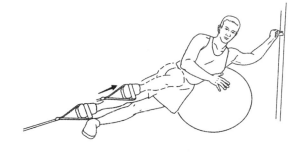

Hip Flexion: Knee-Straight, Single – Side-Lying (Cable)

Flex hip by lifting leg forward, keeping knee straight, torso stable. Repeat with other leg.

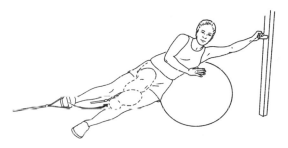

Chapter 4: Arms

The benefit to using the exercise ball when training arms is the ability to emphasize the arm musculature in a functional and specific manner. Clients will find that they need far less resistance to experience gains in strength and muscular development.

Exercises recommended for beginners — This section will help the trainee to become familiar with the movements of the joint being worked and set the foundation for future exercises.

Exercises recommended for intermediates — This section is designed to progress the exerciser to movements that will stress the arms to a greater degree. As with the previous section, care should be taken to progress in a deliberate fashion.

Exercises recommended for advanced — This section is valuable in helping athletes to stress the muscles of the arms in sport specific ways. These exercises are challenging and require a good foundation to be effective.

Beginning — 21 exercises

Intermediate — 20 exercises

Advanced — 7 exercises

Biceps Curl (Dumbbell)

Supported by ball with knees bent, palms forward, curl dumbbells. Do not allow shoulder to flex.

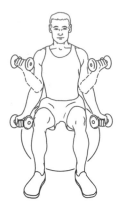

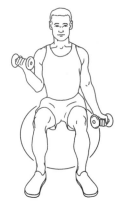

Curl: Alternating (Dumbbell)

Supported by ball with knees slightly bent, curl one dumbbell. Repeat with other arm.

Biceps Curl: Hammer Grip (Dumbbell)

Supported by ball with knees slightly bent, forearms neutral, palms in, curl dumbbells.

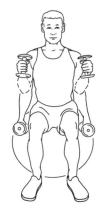

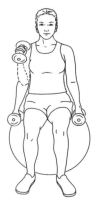

Biceps Curl: Hammer Grip –Alternating (Dumbbell)

Supported by ball with knees slightly bent, palms in, forearms neutral, curl one dumbbell. Repeat with other arm.

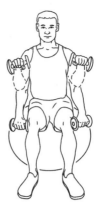

Biceps Curl: Reverse Grip (Dumbbell)

Supported by ball with knees slightly bent. Palms facing rear, curl dumbbells.

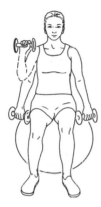

Biceps Curl: Reverse Grip – Alternating (Dumbbell)

Supported by ball with knees slightly bent. Palm facing rear, curl one dumbbell. Repeat with other arm.

Biceps Curl (Dumbbell)

Stand supported by ball with knees slightly bent. Palms facing rear, curl dumbbells, rotating forearms to palms up.

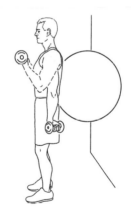

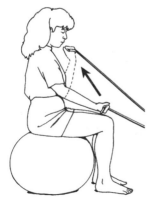

Biceps Curl: Unilateral (Tubing)

With tubing or resistive band secured in door, bend elbow. Can use weights.

Biceps Curl: Sitting (Cable – Low Pulley)

Grasp handles, elbows fully extended. Curl cables.

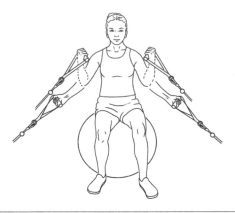

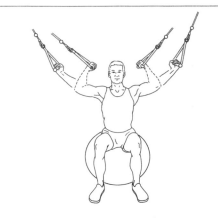

Biceps Curl: Sitting (Cable – High Pulley)

Grasp handles, elbows fully extended, upper arm parallel to floor. Curl cables.

Triceps Kickback (Dumbbell)

Stand with feet staggered, upper body supported by ball, upper arm parallel to floor. Raise dumbbell by extending elbow. Repeat with other arm.

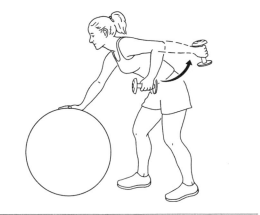

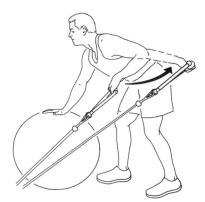

Triceps Kickback (Cable)

Stand with feet staggered, upper body supported by ball, upper arm parallel to floor. Raise cable by extending elbow. Repeat with other arm.

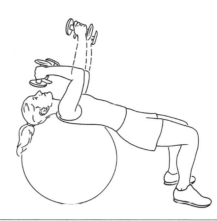

Triceps Extension: Supine (Dumbbell)

Bridge trunk, head and neck supported, upper arms vertical. Raise dumbbells by extending elbows.

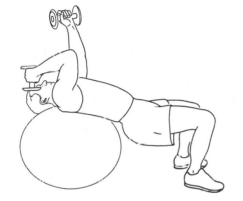

Triceps Extension: Supine – Alternating (Dumbbell)

Bridge trunk, head and neck supported, upper arm vertical. Raise dumbbell by extending elbow. Repeat with other arm.

Triceps Press: Close Grip – Supine (Dumbbell)

Hold dumbbells over chest, elbows in close. Extend elbows.

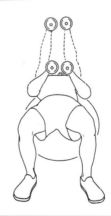

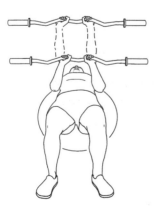

Triceps Press: Close Grip – Supine (EZ Curl Bar)

Hold bar over chest with elbows in close. Extend elbows.

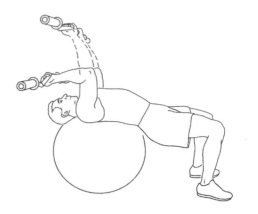

Triceps Extension: Supine (EZ Curl Bar)

Bridge trunk, head and neck supported, upper arms vertical grasping bar. Raise bar by extending elbows.

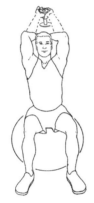

Triceps Extension: Sitting (Dumbbell)

With upper arms vertical, raise dumbbell by extending elbows. Keep feet flat and back straight.

Triceps Extension: Single – Sitting (Dumbbell)

With upper arm vertical, raise dumbbell by extending elbow. Keep feet flat and back straight. Repeat with other arm.

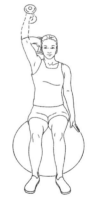

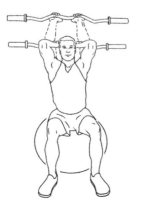

Triceps Extension: Sitting (EZ Curl Bar)

With upper arms vertical, raise bar by extending elbows. Keep feet flat and back straight.

Triceps Push-Up: Close Grip – Kneeling

With hands close, extend elbows by pushing
away from ball. Keep back straight.

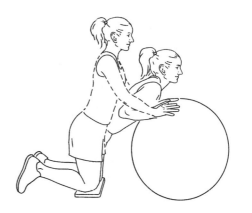

Biceps Curl: Preacher (Dumbbell)

Kneel over ball with elbows fully extended. Curl dumbbells.

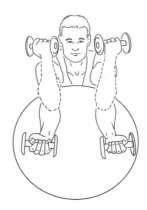

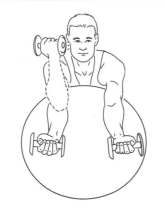

Biceps Curl: Preacher – Alternating (Dumbbell)

Kneel over ball with elbows fully extended. Curl one dumbbell. Repeat with other arm.

Biceps Curl: Preacher – Hammer Grip (Dumbbell)

Kneel over ball with palms facing each other and elbows fully extended. Curl dumbbells.

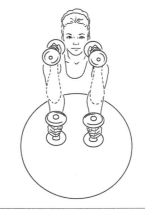

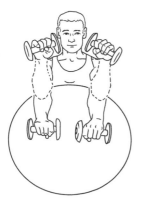

Biceps Curl: Preacher – Reverse Grip (Dumbbell)

Kneel over ball, palms down, elbows fully extended. Curl dumbbells.

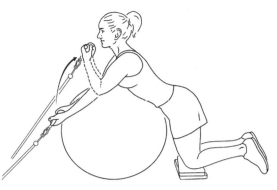

Biceps Curl: Preacher (Cable)

Kneel over ball, elbows fully extended. Curl cable.

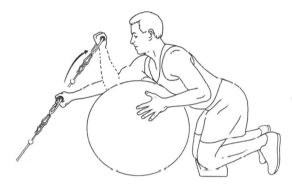

Biceps Curl: Preacher – Single (Cable)

Kneel over ball, elbow fully extended.
Curl cable. Repeat with other arm.

Biceps Curl: Preacher – Reverse Grip (Cable)

Kneel over ball, palms down, elbows
fully extended. Curl cable.

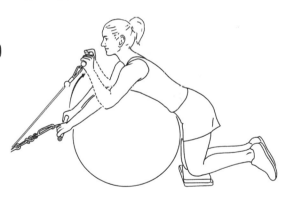

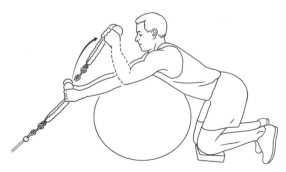

Biceps Curl: Preacher (Cable with Rope)

Kneel over ball, elbows fully extended. Curl cable.

Triceps Extension: Supine (Barbell)

Bridge trunk, head and neck supported, upper arms vertical grasping bar. Raise bar by extending elbows.

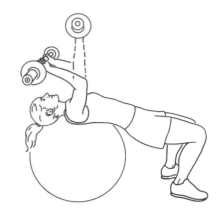

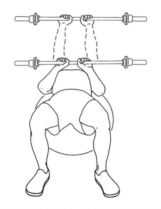

Triceps Press: Close Grip – Supine (Barbell)

Hold bar over chest with elbows in close. Extend elbows.

Triceps Extension: Supine (Cable)

Bridge trunk, with head, neck, and shoulders supported. With upper arms vertical, raise cable by extending elbows.

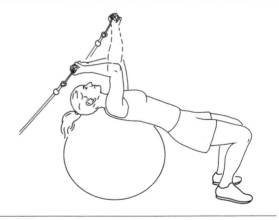

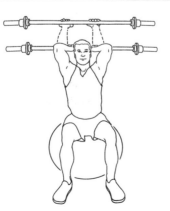

Triceps Extension: Sitting (Barbell)

With upper arms vertical, raise bar by extending elbows. Keep feet flat and back straight.

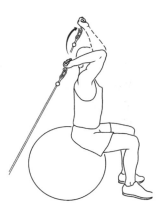

Triceps Extension: Sitting (Cable)

With upper arms vertical, raise cable by extending elbows. Keep feet flat and back straight.

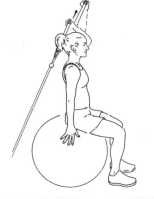

Triceps Extension: Single – Sitting (Cable)

With upper arm vertical, raise cable by extending elbow. Keep feet flat and back straight. Repeat with other arm.

Triceps Extension: Bilateral

With tubing or resistive band secured in door and upper arms parallel to floor, straighten elbows simultaneously.

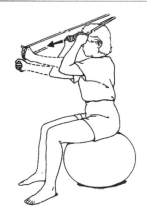

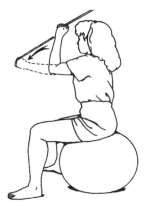

Triceps Extension: Unilateral

With tubing or resistive band secured in door, and upper arm parallel to floor, straighten elbow.

Triceps Extension: Sitting (Smith Machine)

With close grip, allow bar to descend until elbows are at 30° then extend by tightening triceps. Keep back straight.

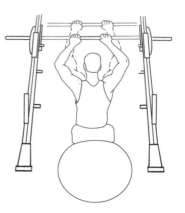

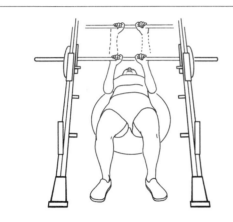

Triceps Press: Close Grip – Supine (Smith Machine)

Hold bar over chest with elbows in close. Extend elbows.

Triceps Push-up: Close Grip – On Toes

With hands close, extend elbow by pushing away from ball. Keep back straight.

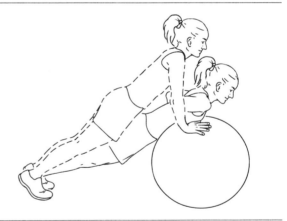

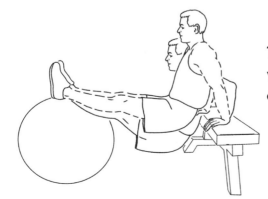

Triceps Dip: Feet on Ball

With feet supported by ball and hands firmly on bench, extend elbows by tightening triceps.

Biceps Curl: Kneeling (Dumbbell)

Kneel on ball with elbows fully extended. Curl dumbbells.

Caution: Spotter advised.

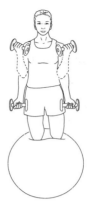

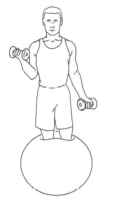

Biceps Curl: Alternating – Kneeling (Dumbbell)

Kneel on ball, elbows fully extended. Curl one dumbbell. Repeat with other arm.

Caution: Spotter advised.

Biceps Curl: Hammer Grip – Kneeling (Dumbbell)

Kneel on ball, palms in, elbows fully extended. Curl dumbbells.

Caution: Spotter advised.

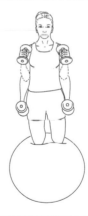

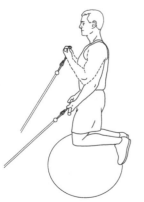

Biceps Curl: Kneeling (Cable)

Kneel on the ball, elbows fully extended, curl cable.

Caution: Spotter advised.

Triceps Press-Down: Kneeling (Cable)

Grasp handle and kneel on ball.
Press cable. Keep back straight.

Caution: Spotter advised.

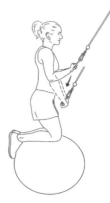

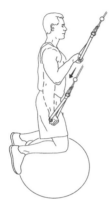

Triceps Press-Down: Single – Kneeling (Cable)

Grasp handle and kneel on ball. Press cable, keep back straight and opposite arm out to side. Repeat with other arm.

Caution: Spotter advised.

Triceps Press-Down: Reverse Grip – Kneeling (Cable)

Grasp handle, palms facing upward, kneel on ball. Press cable. Keep back straight.

Caution: Spotter advised.

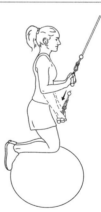

Chapter 5: Chest

The chest muscles can be stressed in a more functional manner when using the exercise ball. All the exercises require the trainee to push and pull in anatomically correct kinematical movement.

Exercises recommended for beginners — This section is designed to help the exerciser become familiar with the correct motions of the chest muscles. It is important to feel the movement and muscles working to experience maximal gains.

Exercises recommended for intermediates — These exercises will help the trainee begin to stress the chest muscles to a greater degree. Again, the benefit of using the ball instead of a bench is that it allows for a greater degree of isolation.

Exercises recommended for advanced — These exercises are very difficult. They will allow the athlete to build on the foundation of the previous two sections. Many situations in sport and activity will call upon the chest muscles to work while in a dynamic situation. These exercises will help to train the athlete for that specific purpose.

Beginning — 12 exercises

Intermediate — 18 exercises

Advanced — 8 exercises

Wall Push-Up: Double Arm (Gymball)

Stand away from wall with both hands supporting a gymball on the wall. Perform a push-up.

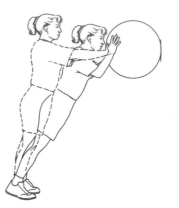

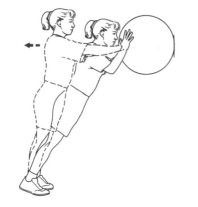

Wall Push-Up Plus: Double Arm (Gymball)

Stand away from wall with both hands supporting a gymball on the wall. Perform a push-up. Give an extra push at end to bring shoulder blades forward on rib cage.

Push-Up from Mid-Thigh: Prone

Roll forward until ball rests under thighs. Perform push-up. Keep back straight.

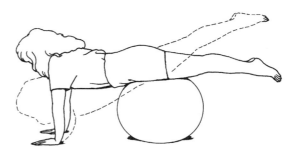

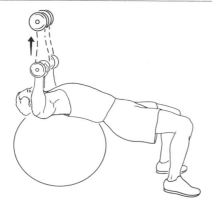

Press (Dumbbell)

Press dumbbells over chest while maintaining bridge.

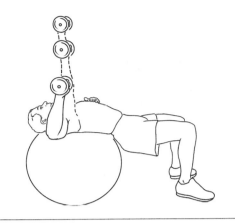

Press Plus: Single (Dumbbell)

Press dumbbell over chest and protract shoulder at end while maintaining bridge. Repeat with other arm.

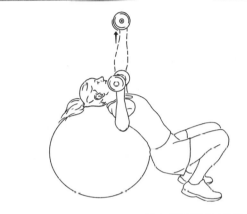

Press: Incline (Dumbbell)

Press dumbbells over head while keeping hips low.

Fly (Dumbbell)

Bring dumbbells toward midline, at chest level, using a hugging motion and maintaining bridge.

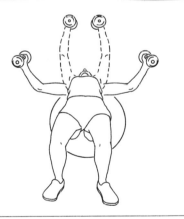

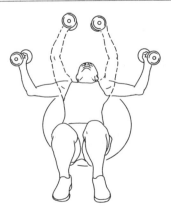

Fly: Incline (Dumbbell)

Bring dumbbells toward midline, chest level using a hugging motion and keeping hips low.

Fly: Sitting (Dumbbell)

With arms slightly bent, bring dumbbells toward midline, chest level.

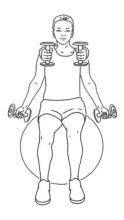

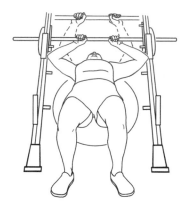

Press: Medium Grip (Smith Machine)

Press bar over chest while maintaining bridge.

Press: Wide Grip (Smith Machine)

Press bar over chest while maintaining bridge.

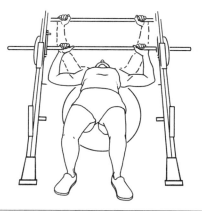

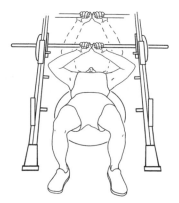

Press: Narrow Grip (Smith Machine)

Press bar over chest while maintaining bridge.

Chest Fly: High / Low – Two-Arm (Tubing)

Arms out from sides at head level, move hands in front of shoulders, and down to hip level.

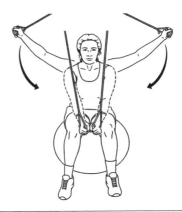

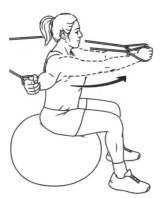

Chest Fly: Low / High – Two-Arm (Tubing)

Arms out from sides at hip level, move hands in front of shoulders, and up to head level.

Chest Press: Two-Arm (Tubing)

Hold tubing in front of shoulders, thumbs in, extend arms forward.

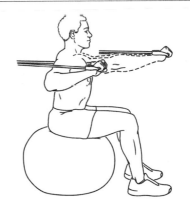

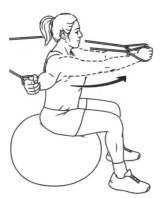

Chest Fly: Two-Arm (Tubing)

Arms out from sides at chest level, move hands in front of shoulders and forward.

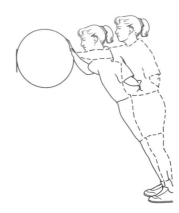

Wall Push-Up: Single Arm (Gymball)

Stand away from wall, one hand supporting
a gymball on the wall. Perform a push-up.

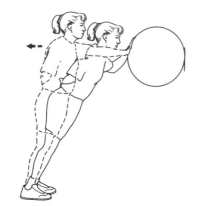

Wall Push-Up Plus: Single Arm (Gymball)

Stand away from wall with one hand supporting
a gymball on the wall, other hand behind back.
Perform a push-up. Give an extra push at end
to bring shoulder blades forward on rib cage.

Push-Up from Shins: Prone

Roll forward until ball rests under shins.
Perform push-up. Keep back straight.

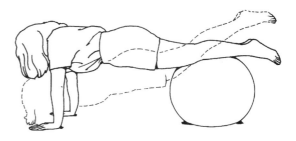

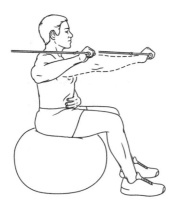

Chest Press: One-Arm (Tubing)

Hold tubing in front of shoulder, thumb in,
other hand on abdomen, extend arm forward.
Keep hips still. Repeat with other arm.

Chest Fly: One-Arm (Tubing)

One arm out from side at chest level, other hand on abdomen, sweep arm toward midline in front of body. Keep hips still. Repeat with other arm.

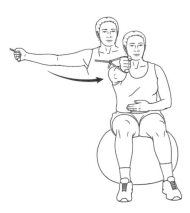

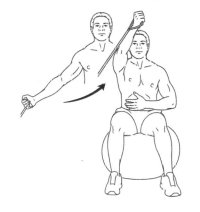

Chest Fly: Low / High – One-Arm (Tubing)

One arm out from side at hip level, other hand on abdomen, sweep arm toward midline in front of body and up to head level. Keep hips still. Repeat with other arm.

Chest Fly: High / Low – One-Arm (Tubing)

One arm out from side at head level, other hand on abdomen, sweep arm toward midline in front of body and down to hip level. Keep hips still. Repeat with other arm.

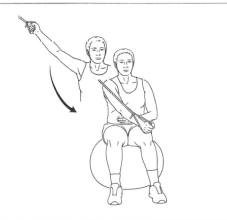

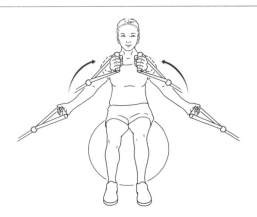

Fly: Sitting (Cable)

Grasp cables with arms slightly bent and bring arms toward midline, chest level.

Fly: Single – Sitting (Cable)

Grasp cable with arm slightly bent and bring arm toward midline, chest level. Repeat with other arm.

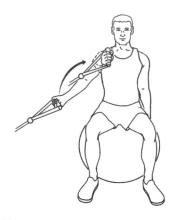

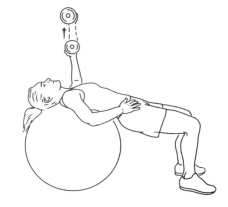

Press: Single (Dumbbell)

Press dumbbell over chest while maintaining bridge. Repeat with other arm.

Press: Incline – Single (Dumbbell)

Press dumbbell over head while keeping hips low. Repeat with other arm.

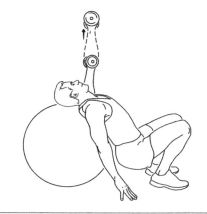

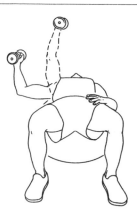

Fly: Single (Dumbbell)

Bring dumbbell toward midline, chest level using a hugging motion and maintaining bridge. Repeat with other arm.

Fly: Single – Incline (Dumbbell)

Bring dumbbell toward midline, chest level using hugging motion and keeping hips low. Repeat with other arm.

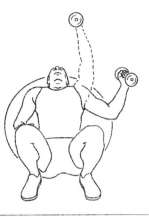

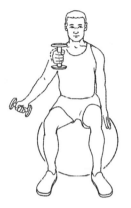

Fly: Single – Sitting (Dumbbell)

With arm slightly bent, bring dumbbell toward midline, chest level. Repeat with other arm.

Press: Medium Grip (Barbell)

Press bar over chest while maintaining bridge.

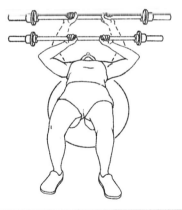

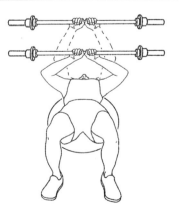

Press: Narrow Grip (Barbell)

Press bar over chest while maintaining bridge. Keep elbows out.

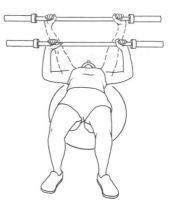

Press: Wide Grip (Barbell)

Press bar over chest while maintaining bridge.

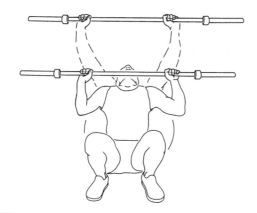

Press: Incline (Barbell)

Press bar over chest while keeping hips low.

Fly: Kneeling (Dumbbell)

With arms slightly bent bring dumbbells to chest level.

Caution: Spotter advised.

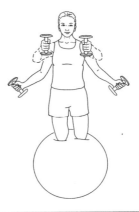

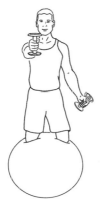

Fly: Alternating – Kneeling (Dumbbell)

With arms slightly bent bring one dumbbell toward midline, chest level. Repeat with other arm.

Caution: Spotter advised.

Fly: Kneeling (Cable)

Grasp cables with arms slightly bent and bring arms toward midline, chest level.

Caution: Spotter advised.

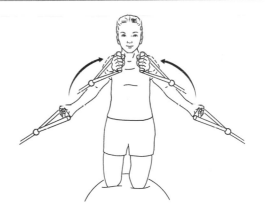

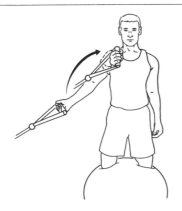

Fly: Single (Cable)

Grasp cable with arm slightly bent and bring arm toward midline, chest level. Repeat with other arm.

Caution: Spotter advised.

Walkout Foam Roller Push-Up (Gymball)

Hands on foam roller, walk-roll out to {hips, knees, shins, toes}. Perform push-up.

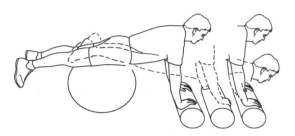

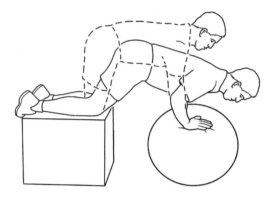

Hands on Ball: Push-Up

Kneel on surface level with top of ball. Place hands on ball. Maintain shoulders over ball. Perform a push-up.

Push-Up from Toes: Prone

Roll forward until ball rests under toes. Perform push-up. Keep back straight.

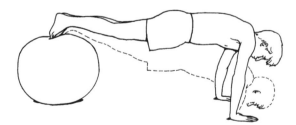

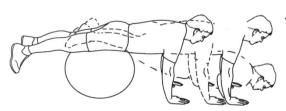

Walkout: with Push-Up (Gymball)

Walk-roll out to shins. Perform push-up.

Chapter 6: Back

This section will benefit the exerciser by allowing the motions of the back muscles to follow a pure line of movement. Do to the inherent instability of the ball, all of these exercises must be done with proper form and posture to stimulate the back muscles. If not, very little gain will be seen.

Exercises recommended for beginners — In conjunction with the trunk and abdominals; these exercises will help to increase better postural strength and awareness. The beginning exercises will help the trainee to focus on the various pulling motions of the back muscles.

Exercises recommended for intermediates — These exercises can be used for strength as well as muscle building. They will help to increase the total strength of the core.

Exercises recommended for advanced — Athletes can benefit greatly from this section. Many sports activities call upon the trainee to pull in an unstable environment. This section will help to familiarize the person with those types of situations.

Beginning — 17 exercises

Intermediate — 11 exercises

Advanced — 5 exercises

Scapular Retraction: Kneeling

Bend arms and lift, pulling shoulder blades together.

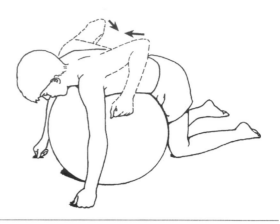

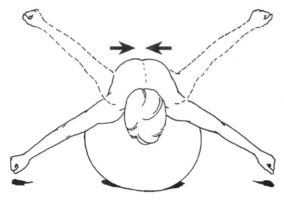

Butterflies: Kneeling

Kneeling on floor with stomach over ball, extend arms and lift to pull shoulder blades together.

Scapular Retraction: Unilateral

With tubing or resistive band secured in door and other end looped around upper arm, pull shoulder blade toward spine.

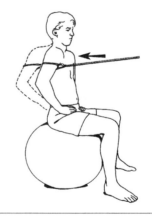

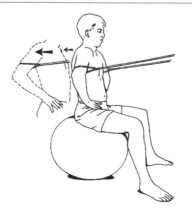

Scapular Retraction: Bilateral

With tubing or resistive band secured in door and ends looped around upper arms, pull shoulder blades together.

Abduction: Bilateral

Using tubing or resistive band, lift arms straight out until parallel to floor.

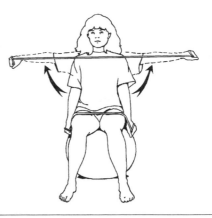

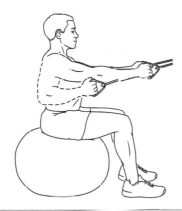

Row: Two-Arm (Tubing)

With arms reaching forward, pull tubing to sides of chest, palms in or up.

Fly: Reverse – Two-Arm (Tubing)

With arms reaching forward, pull tubing from midline out to sides at shoulder level.

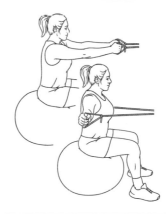

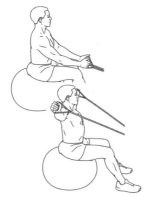

Fly: Reverse – Low / High, Two-Arm (Tubing)

With arms reaching forward and down, pull tubing up and out.

Fly: Reverse – High / Low, Two-Arm (Tubing)

With arms reaching forward and up, pull tubing down and out.

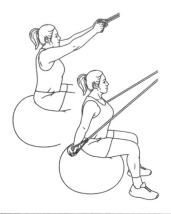

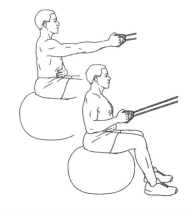

Row: One-Arm (Tubing)

With one arm forward, other hand on abdomen, pull tubing to side of chest, palm in or up. Keep hips still. Repeat with other arm.

Fly: Reverse – One-Arm (Tubing)

With one arm reaching forward, other hand on abdomen, pull tubing from midine of chest out to side of body. Keep hips still. Repeat with other arm.

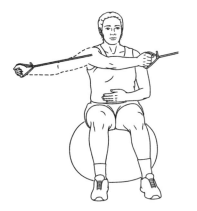

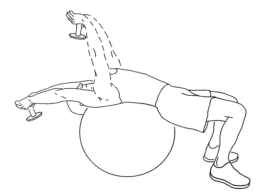

Pullover (Dumbbell)

Pull dumbbell over chest, keeping elbows straight, trunk bridged.

Row: Prone (Dumbbell)

Pull weights to sides, palms facing floor.

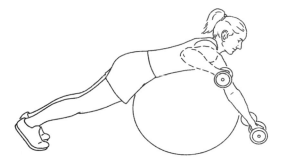

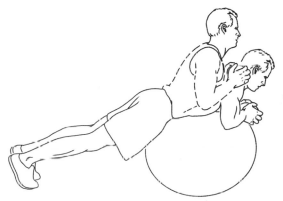

Extension: Prone (Dumbbell)

Hold dumbbell in front of chest and extend low back.

Row: Sitting – Bent Over (Dumbbell)

Pull weights to sides, palms facing each other.

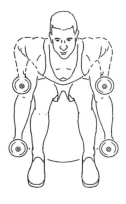

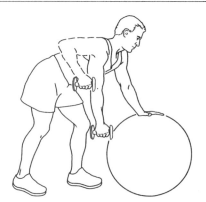

Row: Single (Dumbbell)

With feet staggered, arm supported, pull weight to side of chest, keeping elbow close. Keep back straight. Repeat with other arm.

Row: Reverse Grip Single (Dumbbell)

With feet staggered, arm supported, pull weight to side of chest, palm forward. Keep back straight. Repeat with other arm.

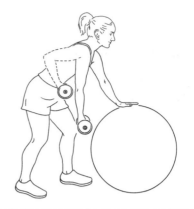

Row: Close Grip – Sitting (Cable)

Pull weight to top of abdomen, keeping back straight.

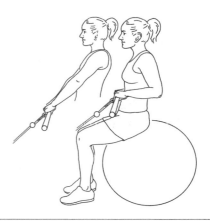

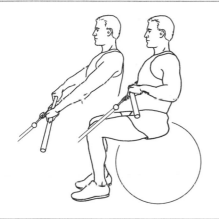

Row: Medium Grip – Sitting (Cable)

Pull weight to top of abdomen, keeping back straight.

Row: Wide Grip – Sitting (Cable)

Pull weight to top of abdomen, keeping back straight.

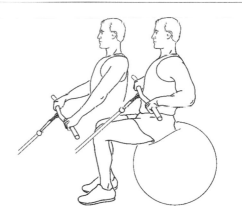

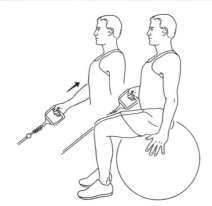

Row: Single – Sitting (Cable)

Pull weight to the side of the abdomen, keeping back straight. Repeat with other arm.

Row: Reverse Grip – Single, Sitting (Cable)

With palm facing upward, pull weight to the side of the abdomen, keeping back straight. Repeat with other arm.

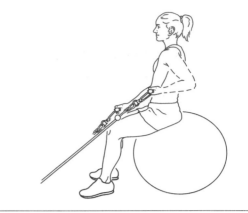

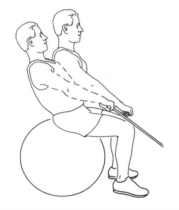

Extension: Sitting (Cable)

Hold cable in front of chest and extend low back.

Pull-Down: Wide Grip – Sitting (Cable)

Pull weight to top of chest.
Keep low back arched.

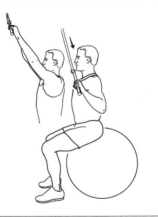

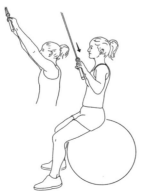

Pull-Down: Close Grip – Sitting (Cable)

Pull weight to top of chest. Keep low back arched.

Pull-Down: Reverse Grip – Sitting (Cable)

With palms facing body, pull weight down
to top of chest. Keep low back arched.

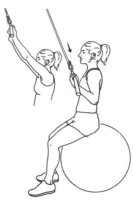

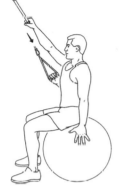

Pull-Down: Single – Sitting (Cable)

Pull weight to side of chest. Keep low
back arched. Repeat with other arm.

Pull-Down: Reverse Grip – Single, Sitting (Cable)

With palm facing body, pull weight
down to side of chest. Keep low back
arched. Repeat with other arm.

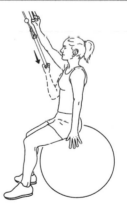

Pullover (EZ Curl Bar)

Pull bar over chest, keeping elbows straight, trunk bridged.

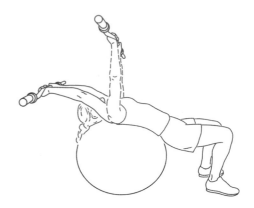

Pullover (Barbell)

Pull bar over chest, keeping elbows straight, trunk bridged.

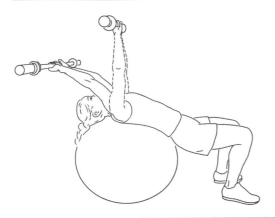

Pullover (Cable)

Pull cable over chest, keeping elbows straight, trunk bridged.

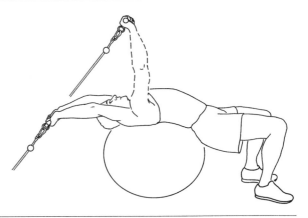

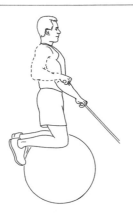

Row: Kneeling (Cable)

Pull weight to top of abdomen, keeping back straight.

Caution: Spotter advised.

Pull-Down: Kneeling (Cable)

Pull weight to top of chest. Keep back straight.

Caution: Spotter advised.

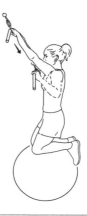

Chapter 7: Shoulders

As with several of the previous chapters, trainees will realize that less resistance will be necessary to feel the stress on the shoulder muscles. It is very important to stimulate all portions of the shoulder in order to create a stable and healthy joint. This section will allow the exerciser to do just that.

Exercises recommended for beginners — This section offers the exerciser the chance to become proficient in the basic motions of the shoulder joint. The trainee should see better postural habits if they perform the exercises in this section correctly.

Exercises recommended for intermediates — This section begins to move the trainee to exercises that will help to increase muscularity. As with the previous section, strict attention to form is a must.

Exercises recommended for advanced — This section is designed to further enhance the strength and stability of the shoulder joint in a dynamic environment.

Beginning — 17 exercises

Intermediate — 11 exercises

Advanced — 5 exercises

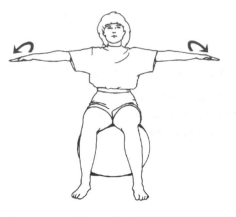

Arm Circles: Bilateral

With arms straight out from sides, make forward circles.

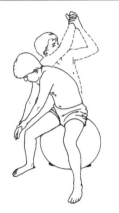

PNF: Diagonal Chop 1 – Sitting

Grasp wrist and perform an upward reach across body. Keep palm facing toward you. Return to start, maintaining grasp.

PNF: Diagonal Chop 2 – Sitting

Grasp wrist and perform an upward reach across body. Keep thumb pointing behind you. Return to start, maintaining grasp.

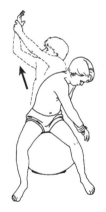

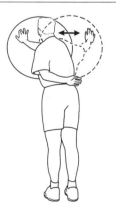

Gymball on Wall: Side to Side

Stand away from wall with right hand supporting a ball on the wall. Lean into ball and move ball side to side.

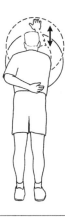

Gymball on Wall: Up and Down

Stand away from wall with one hand supporting a ball on the wall. Lean into ball and move ball up and down.

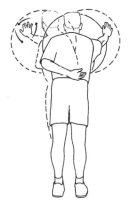

Gymball on Wall: Clockwise / Counterclockwise

Stand away from wall with one hand supporting a ball on the wall. Lean into ball and move ball in circles clockwise, then counterclockwise.

Raise: Side (Dumbbell)

Back straight, raise dumbbells from sides.

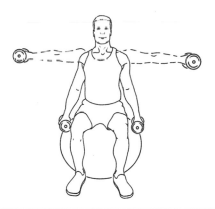

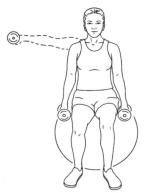

Raise: Side – Single (Dumbbell)

Back straight, raise one dumbbell from side. Repeat with other arm.

Press (Dumbbell)

Back straight, press dumbbells over head.

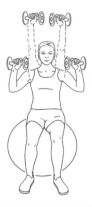

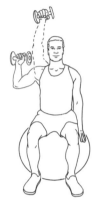

Press: Single (Dumbbell)

Back straight, press dumbbell over head. Repeat with other arm.

Raise: Front (Dumbbell)

Back straight, raise dumbbell forward.

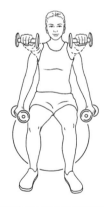

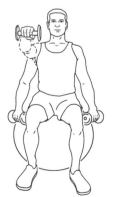

Raise: Front – Single (Dumbbell)

Back straight, raise one dumbbell forward. Repeat with other arm.

Fly: Rear – Prone (Dumbbell)

Back straight, arm slightly bent, raise dumbbells to shoulder level.

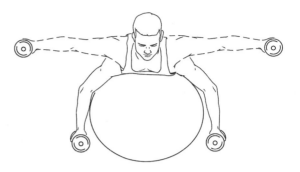

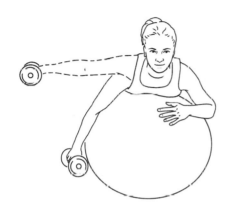

Fly: Rear – Single, Prone (Dumbbell)

Back straight, arms slightly bent, raise one dumbbell to shoulder level. Repeat with other arm.

External Rotation: Sitting (Dumbbell)

Elbows steady, rotate forearms out.

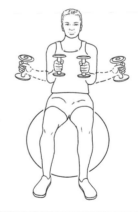

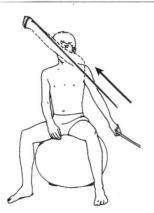

PNF: Diagonal 1 Flexion

With tubing secured low in door and arm at side, pull up and across body. Keep palm facing behind you. Can use resistive band or weights.

PNF: Diagonal 2 Flexion

With tubing secured low in door and held by arm on opposite side, bring up and across body. Keep thumb pointing upward. Can use resistive band or weights.

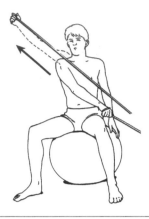

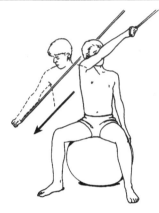

PNF: Diagonal 1 Extension

With tubing secured high in door and held by arm on opposite side, bring down and across body. Keep palm facing toward you. Can use resistive band or weights.

PNF: Diagonal 2 Extension

With tubing secured high in door and held by same-side arm, bring arm down and across body. Keep thumb pointing behind you. Can use resistive band or weights.

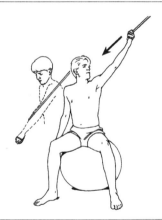

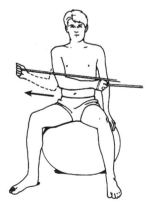

Shoulder External Rotation

With tubing or resistive band secured in door, rotate arm away. Keep elbow bent at right angle.

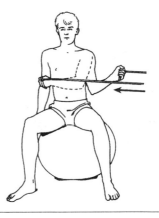

Shoulder Internal Rotation

With tubing or resistive band secured in door, rotate arm toward you. Keep elbow bent at right angle.

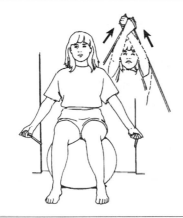

PNF: Diagonal 1 Flexion – Bilateral

With tubing secured low in door, bring arms up and across body. Keep palms facing toward you. Can use resistive band or weights.

PNF: Diagonal 2 Flexion – Bilateral

With tubing secured low in door and arms crossed, reach above head, uncrossing arms. Keep thumbs pointing up. Can use resistive band or weights.

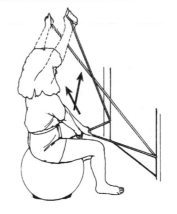

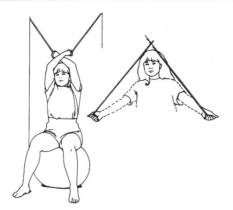

PNF: Diagonal 1 Extension – Bilateral

With tubing secured high in door and arms crossed, reach down and away, uncrossing arms. Can use resistive band or weights.

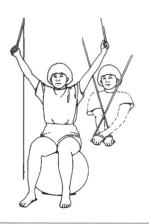

PNF: Diagonal 2 Extension – Bilateral

With tubing secured high in door and arms out, bring both arms down, crossing in front. Can use resistive band or weights.

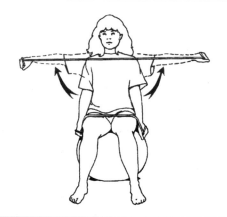

Abduction: Bilateral

Using tubing or resistive band, lift arms straight out until parallel to floor.

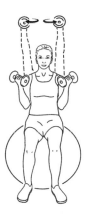

Press: "Arnold" (Dumbbell)

Back straight, palms facing backward, press weights over head, rotating to palms in.

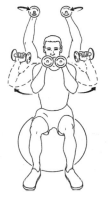

Press: "4 Point"

Palms in, elbows in, swing elbows out from sides, then press weights over head, palms forward. Rotate to palms in and return.

Press (Cable)

Back straight, press cable over head.

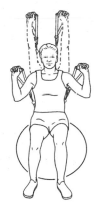

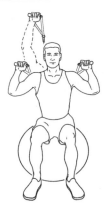

Press: Alternating (Cable)

Back straight, press cable over head. Repeat with other arm.

Press: Front (Barbell)

Back straight, press barbell over head.

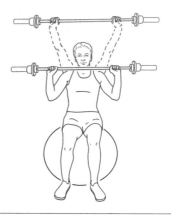

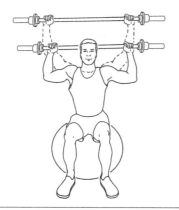

Press: Rear (Barbell)

Back straight, press barbell over head.

Raise: Side (Cable)

Back straight, raise cable from sides.

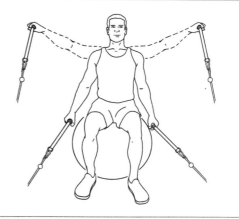

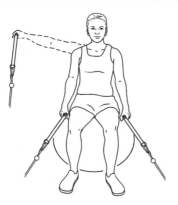

Raise: Side – Single (Cable)

Back straight, raise cable from side. Repeat with other arm.

Raise: Front (Cable)

Back straight, raise cable forward.

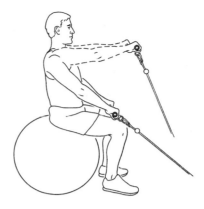

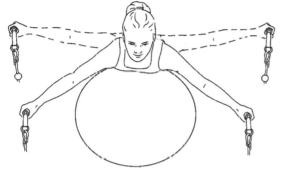

Fly: Rear – Prone (Cable)

Back straight, arms slightly bent, raise cables in line with shoulders.

Fly: Rear – Single, Prone (Cable)

Back straight, arms slightly bent, raise cable in line with shoulder. Repeat with other arm.

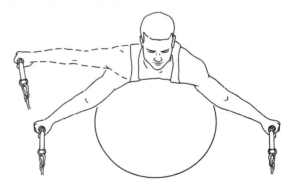

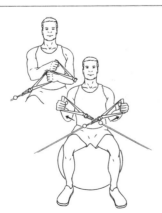

External Rotation: Sitting (Cable)

Elbows steady, rotate forearms out.

Internal Rotation: Sitting (Cable)

Elbow steady, rotate forearm toward
trunk. Repeat with other arm.

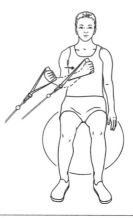

Gymball on Wall: Partner Resistance

Stand away from wall. Support ball with one hand, other hand behind back. Resist as partner attempts to push your arm up. Don't let your arm move. Repeat with other arm.

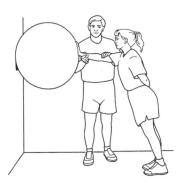

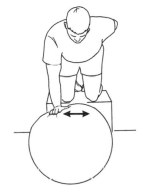

Hand on Ball: Side to Side

Kneel on surface level with top of ball. Place one hand on ball, other hand behind back. Maintain shoulders over ball. Move ball side to side. Repeat with other arm.

Hand on Ball: Front to Back

Kneel on surface level with top of ball. Place one hand on ball, other hand behind back. Maintain shoulders over ball. Move ball forward to back. Repeat with other arm.

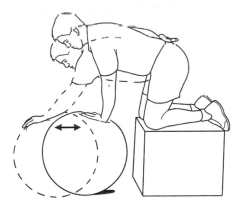

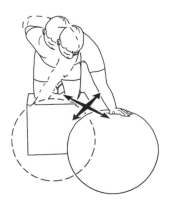

Hand on Ball: Diagonal

Kneel on surface level with top of ball. Place one hand on ball, other hand behind back. Maintain shoulders over ball. Move ball in diagonal pattern, forward to back, alternating directions. Repeat with other arm.

Hand on Ball: Circle – Clockwise / Counterclockwise

Kneel on surface level with top of ball. Place one hand on ball, other hand behind back. Maintain shoulders over ball. Move ball in circles clockwise, then counterclockwise. Repeat with other arm.

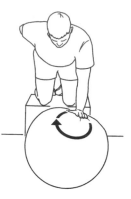

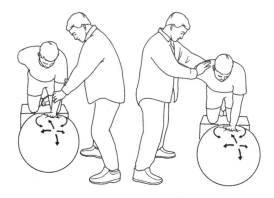

Hand on Ball: Partner Resist

Kneel on surface, level with top of ball. Place one hand on ball, other hand behind back. Maintain shoulders over ball. Resist arm movement as partner attempts to push you forward, backward, side to side, in circle at arm, shoulder, or trunk. Repeat with other arm.

Raise: Side-Lying

With trunk supported, raise dumbbell toward ceiling. Repeat with other arm.

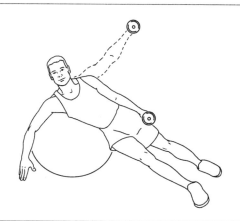

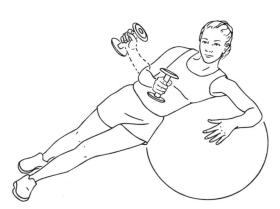

External Rotation: Single – Side-Lying (Dumbbell)

Elbow steady, rotate forearm out. Repeat with other arm.

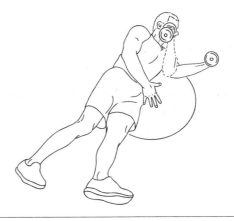

Internal Rotation: Side-Lying (Dumbbell)

Elbow steady, rotate forearm toward trunk. Repeat with other arm.

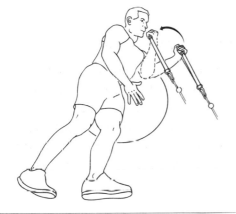

Internal Rotation: Side-Lying (Cable)

Elbow steady, rotate forearm toward trunk. Repeat with other arm.

External Rotation: Single – Side-Lying (Cable)

Elbow steady, rotate forearm out. Repeat with other arm.

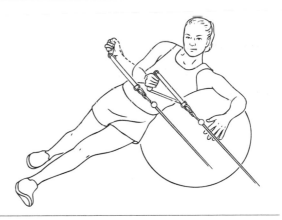

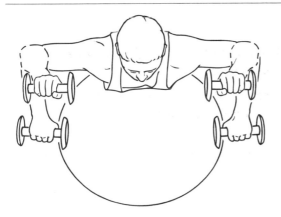

External Rotation: Prone

Back straight, shoulders and elbows at 90-90, raise forearms to horizontal.

Chapter 8: Combinations

This chapter is not for beginners. These exercises are to be performed to provide a fun and unique experience to traditional muscle specific exercises. This section can also be used to stimulate the cardiovascular system and hence help in burning more calories.

Exercises recommended for intermediates and advanced — This is one of the author's favorite sections in that it calls into play all of the systems that make ball training fun and challenging. You will need balance, stability, strength, and endurance to perform the exercises in this section to their greatest potential. The exercises in this chapter can be performed as a complete workout.

Intermediate / Advanced — 24 exercises

Squat Supported / Shoulder Press

Press dumbbells while rising.

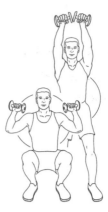

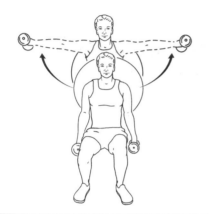

Squat Supported / Side Raise

Raise dumbbells to side while rising.

Squat Supported / Triceps Extension

Extend elbows while rising.

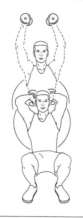

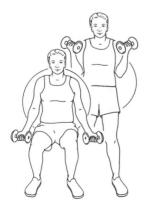

Squat Supported / Biceps Curl

Curl dumbbell while rising.

Squat Supported / Chest Fly

Bring dumbbells toward midline,
chest level while rising.

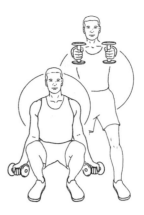

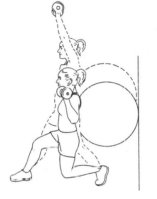

Squat-Split Supported / Shoulder Press

Press dumbbells while rising.
Repeat with feet switched.

Squat-Split Supported / Side Raise

From squat, raise dumbbells while
rising. Repeat with feet switched.

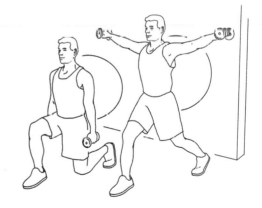

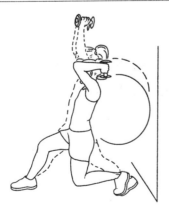

Squat-Split Supported / Triceps Extension

Extend elbows while rising.
Repeat with feet switched.

Squat-Split Supported / Biceps Curl: Single

Curl dumbbell while rising. Repeat
with other arm, feet switched.

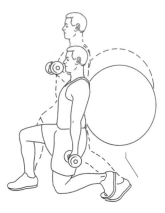

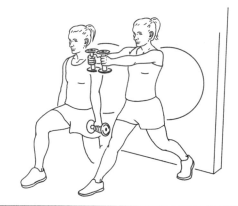

Squat-Split Supported / Chest Fly

Bring dumbbells toward midline, chest level
while rising. Repeat with feet switched.

Shoulder Press / Leg Press

Press dumbbells while rolling ball away from feet.

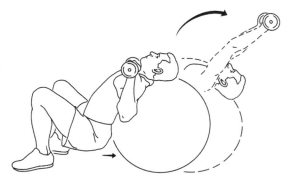

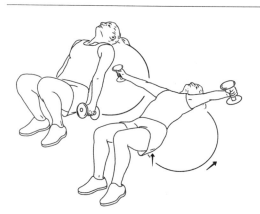

Side Raise / Leg Press

Raise dumbbells while rolling ball away from feet.

Triceps Extension / Leg Press

Extend elbows while rolling ball away from feet.

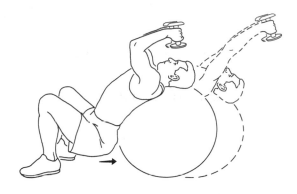

Biceps Curl / Leg Press

Curl dumbbells while rolling ball away from feet.

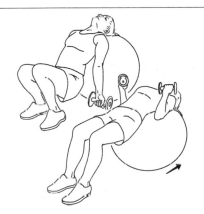

Chest Fly / Leg Press

Bring dumbbells toward midline, chest level, rolling ball away from feet.

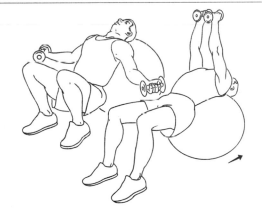

Pullover / Leg Press

Pull dumbbells forward while rolling ball away from feet.

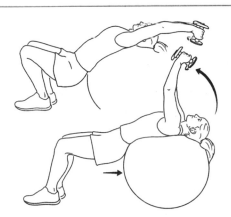

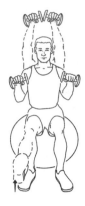

Shoulder Press
with Alternating Knee Extension

Press dumbbells over head and extend
one knee. Repeat with other leg.

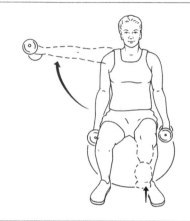

Side Raise / Knee Extension: Single

Raise dumbbell and extend opposite
knee. Repeat with other arm and leg.

Side Raise with Alternating Knee Extension

Raise dumbbells out from sides and extend
one knee. Repeat with other leg.

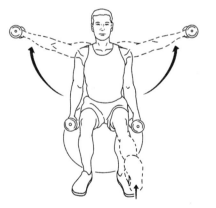

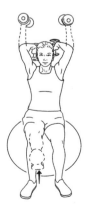

Triceps Extension
with Alternating Knee Extension

Extend elbows and extend one
knee. Repeat with other leg.

Triceps Extension / Knee Extension: Single

Extend elbow and extend knee on the opposite side. Repeat with other arm and leg.

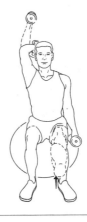

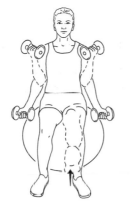

Biceps Curl
with Alternating Knee Extension

Curl dumbbells and extend one knee. Repeat with other leg.

Biceps Curl / Knee Extension: Single

Curl dumbbell and extend opposite knee. Repeat with other arm and leg.

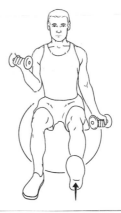

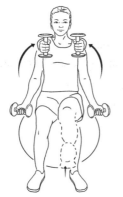

Chest Fly with Alternating Knee Extension

Bring dumbbells toward midline, chest level, and extend one knee. Repeat with other leg.

About VHI

Visual Health Information (VHI) is the leading publisher of reproducible exercise tools. VHI has been producing exercise collections for the rehabilitation and fitness markets since 1980.

VHI produces reproducible exercise cards and computer software. VHI has over 35 different exercise collections. These collections include exercises for Outpatient Physical Therapy, Geriatrics, Pediatrics, Fitness, Strength & Conditioning, Pre/Postnatal, Speech, Pulmonary Rehab and much more.

The content for the Exercise Idea book series is derived from the over 9,000 exercise images in the VHI exercise database. These books are designed to show you the wide range of exercises that can be used for specific purposes.

To view all the VHI offerings and collections, visit **www.vhikits.com,** or call **1-800-356-0709.**